T0324339

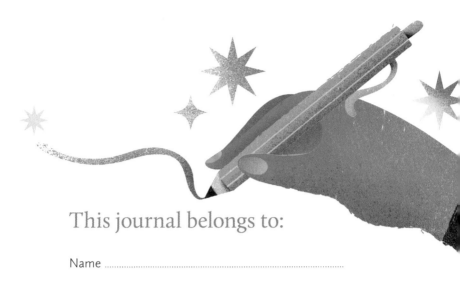

This journal belongs to:

Name ....

Email ....

Telephone ....

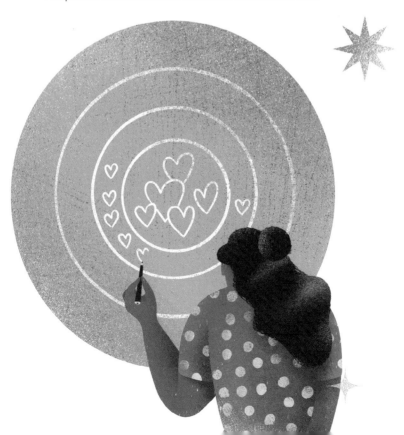

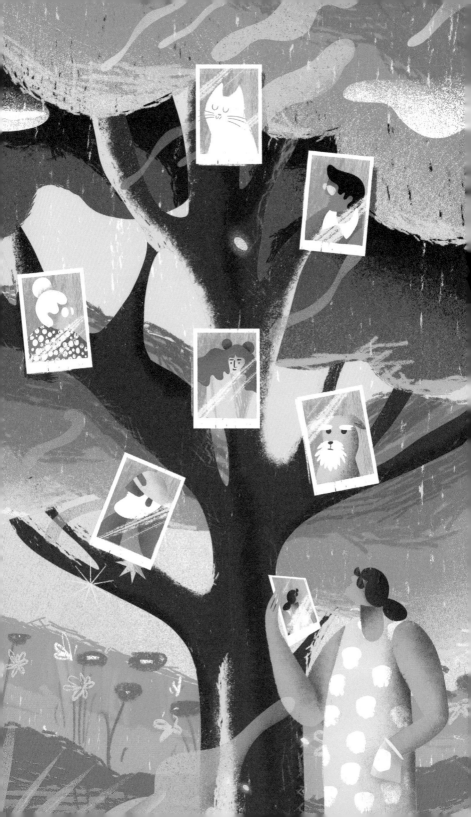

Breathe

Connection

JOURNAL

AMMONITE
PRESS

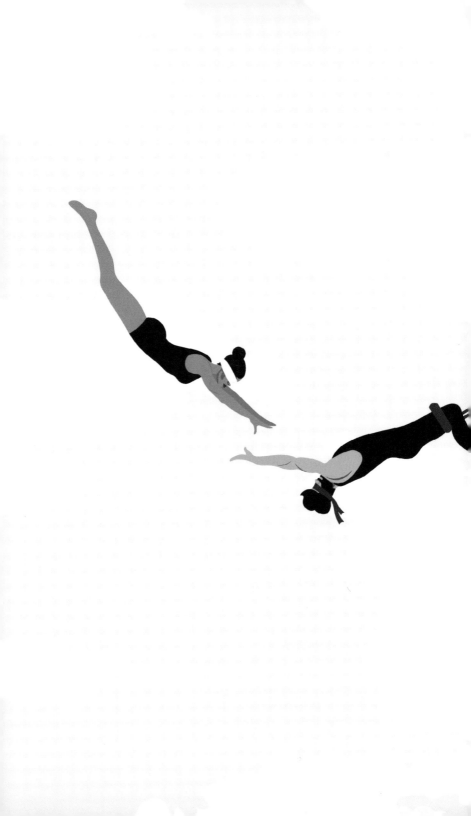

Connection

Despite what the novels and films might lead you to believe, few people are intuitively great at relationships. They take work, commitment and compassion. But even then, personal connections are a complex mix of love, trust, disappointment, affection, acceptance, restriction, loyalty and betrayal. It can be heartening to realise that everyone, no matter the picture presented to the outside world, struggles in the face of the challenges that can arise when you try to build and maintain meaningful connections.

Whether it's family, partners, friendships or even strangers – relationships are a fertile ground for growth and emotional development. Every interaction with someone else is an opportunity to listen more and relate to people in a fresh, empathetic way.

And that's where this journal comes in. With guided exercises, prompts and tips, it's your chance to better understand yourself and others, to foster hope, forgiveness, passion and patience. Use it to develop skills to help you open channels of communication and embrace contentment, however you choose to connect.

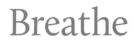

Breathe
breathemagazine.com

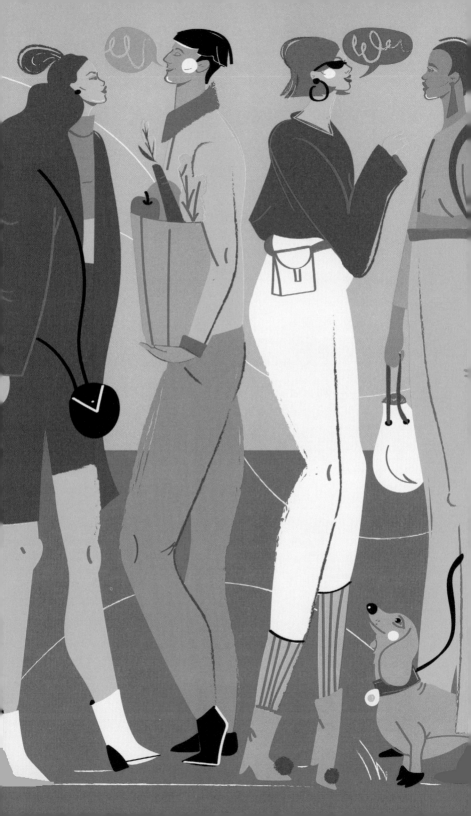

Contents

Power of the breath

How bringing conscious awareness to inhaling and exhaling could provide more than a lungful of air

There's a type of breathwork that's gaining in popularity around the world – and it's not the kind of meditative pranayama often found in yoga classes. Although the practice, known as conscious connected breathing, puts the body into a calmer state – just as pranayama does – advocates say it has the potential to do much more, such as release long-held trauma and remove barriers to the authentic self.

On the surface, conscious connected breathing (or CCB, as it's known) is a tool, and a simple one at that. It is exactly as described – consciously breathing, with no pauses between the inhale and exhale. Forms of it have been used in various modalities, by differing types of practitioners. And like any tool, its applications are as varied as the people using it.

Origins of the practice
It dates back to the 1970s, when it was first used for two techniques known as holotropic breathwork and rebirthing. People have reported varied experiences with these, depending on the practitioner who's running the session. Rebirthing often involves a fast inhale and exhale through the nose. Although both techniques are still in use today, conscious connected breathing has emerged from the older practices and been developed by new practitioners. Although there are countless ways to run a session, just as there are with yoga, many of the newer practices use a wide, open-mouthed inhale, using the diaphragm, into both belly and chest, while the exhale is a simple letting go.

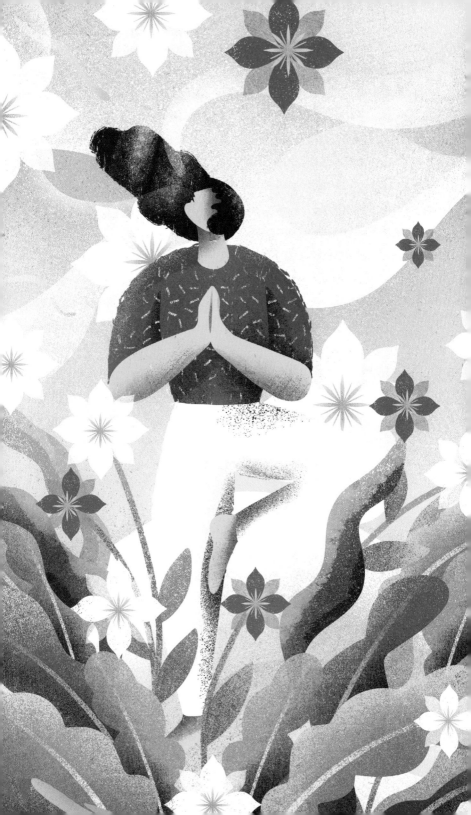

Place of safety

This was the type of workshop that Nicola Price experienced 11 years ago, when she gave connected breathwork a go. 'For the first time, I felt held enough,' she says, and the safety she experienced during the session enabled her to release childhood trauma from her body. 'There was so much locked into my hips from years ago,' she says. 'And I'd had absolutely no idea.'

After that initial session, Nicola – whose background lies in corporate training – went on an exploration of CCB. This led to the creation in 2012 of a programme called Inspirational Breathing, which trains people using her own approach to breathwork. 'I wanted to explore more of the tools around to support it,' she explains. She uses elements of touch, toning, movement, affirmations and visualisation. And she's constantly evolving her practice. 'I've always been an experimenter and an explorer. I put everything through its paces with myself first.'

Nicola suggests a longer inhale than exhale, using a pattern of inhaling for two counts and exhaling for one. She claims rapid breathing, using a short, sharp inhale and a longer exhale, can cause hyperventilation, leading to low levels of carbon dioxide in the bloodstream. There have been anecdotal reports that this can contribute to a syndrome called tetany, which causes muscle twitching and cramps, especially in the hands. 'It puts [some] people off breathwork, and you really don't need it to happen,' says Nicola. 'It's why I give the ratio of inhaling for two counts with "I am", and exhaling with "here" for one.'

Letting go

Brighton-based teacher Jasmine Fish is also an advocate of CCB. She discovered it three years ago and says it's changed her life. 'I've done a lot of meditation and yoga, I've been on shamanic journeys, and nothing was like this,' is how she describes her first session. 'It was an incredible experience.' In that initial workshop, Jasmine says: 'I experienced amazing visualisations, and then went into this state of really beautiful bliss.' And, as she – like Nicola – went on an exploration of breathwork, she found it had more far-reaching benefits, including alleviating the anxiety that had plagued her for years. 'I used to have a lifelong issue with insomnia, and my practice has led to a vast improvement in the management of that,' she says. 'It's also changed me from feeling constantly anxious to feeling safe, and that's made a major difference to my life.'

Inner connections

How could a breath practice lead to such a boost in mental health, plus release decades-old trauma held within the body? Science is well-versed in the theory behind putting the body into a parasympathetic state – also known as the rest-and-digest nervous system – and this can be achieved with many kinds of conscious breathwork.

But this alone can't explain the other claimed benefits of CCB, and the science behind it isn't yet fully understood. It is, at its essence, experiential, which means that as every participant is different, each person's experience will differ – so it's sensible to proceed carefully. Nicola says that it 'brings you into the present moment and into truth and allows you to explore what's happening physically at a really deep level'.

'When we feel safe enough to expose our shadows, that's when we become free'

Gabby Bernstein

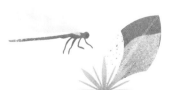

It's personal

As for me, I discovered CCB a few months into the pandemic. My initial caution meant that little happened at first, except that I took 10 distraction-free minutes out of my day to breathe – enough of a bonus in itself. However, as I trusted the practice more, and explored further, I found it drawing all sorts of things out of me, including a heightened self-awareness and understanding. I'm now a convert.

Your breath is under your control, so you can breathe as slowly as you like, for as little or as long as you like. You might attain a state of bliss, find your hips shaking or your spine arching. You might see visions or experience trauma release. Or you might feel nothing. Take your breathwork at a pace comfortable for you and practise as much caution as you wish. You can practise alone but there are plenty of live, often free, breathwork sessions held online. Qualified facilitators of CCB should encourage you to take responsibility for your own practice.

Taking control

Jasmine, who's now a trained CCB facilitator, uses it for any issue she might have. 'If ever things get tough, I'll do a session three or four times a week, and I do a 10-minute practice every day, no matter what,' she says. 'It's helped me storm forward through issues I had for decades and are now completely over. It's changed my outlook and my experience of life so dramatically in such a short period of time... it's been incredibly powerful.'

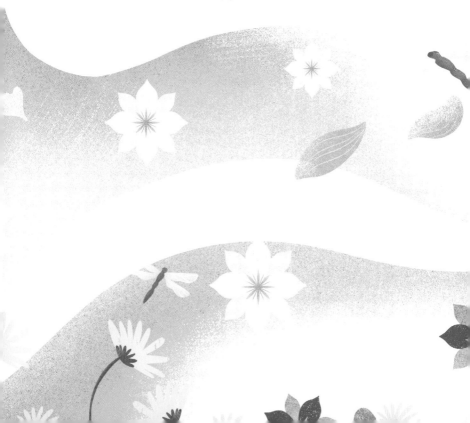

CCB: A BASIC GUIDE

Start with five minutes a day, set the metronome of the breath and start becoming aware.

- Relaxing your jaw, open your mouth very wide.

- Inhale deeply, using your belly and your chest, to the count of two: 'I am.'

- Without a pause, let go as you exhale to the count of one: 'here.'

- Immediately inhale as before, with no pause.

- Continue for five minutes. Repeat every day.

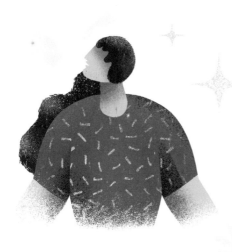

BREATH PRACTICES

1. Holotropic breathwork
Developed in the 1970s by Christina and Stanislav Grof, this is often used as a spiritual practice, with paired participants in a group setting, one 'sitter' and one 'breather'. The breathing is usually very fast and very deep, with little specific guidance from the facilitator, and sessions can last for several hours.

2. Rebirthing
Also developed in the 1970s, rebirthing is another spiritual practice aimed at flooding the body with something founder Leonard Orr called 'Divine Energy', as well as healing early childhood trauma. It uses conscious connected breathing via the nose and can be fast and upper-chest-based rather than diaphragm-focused.

3. Cardiac coherence
This controlled breath technique is theorised to be effective at slowing and stabilising the heartbeat. It involves slow, deep breaths, in for five seconds and out for five seconds. At the very least, it – or any slow, deep, regular breathing – can help lower stress and anxiety and switch your nervous system into a parasympathetic state.

4. Lion's breath
A pranayamic favourite in many a yoga class, often done on hands and knees and great as a reminder never to take yourself too seriously. Take a breath in and, on the exhale, widen your eyes and roll them upwards, while exhaling forcefully as you stick your tongue out, in an energising breath reminiscent of a lion's roar.

5. Wim Hof breathing method
Famed for spending inordinate amounts of time in very cold places, Hof's method is aimed at physiological improvement, such as a boosted immune system, increased energy and better sleep. His daily breath practice is a cycle of 30 to 40 connected breaths. This, combined with exposure to cold and a focused mindset, will, according to his website, provide you with 'a happier, healthier and stronger life'.

Breathwork is contraindicated for several health conditions, including (but not limited to) glaucoma, epilepsy, pregnancy, high blood pressure, aneurysm and diabetes. Please check with a medical professional before embarking on any breathwork practice.

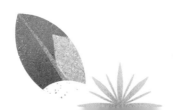
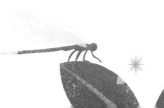

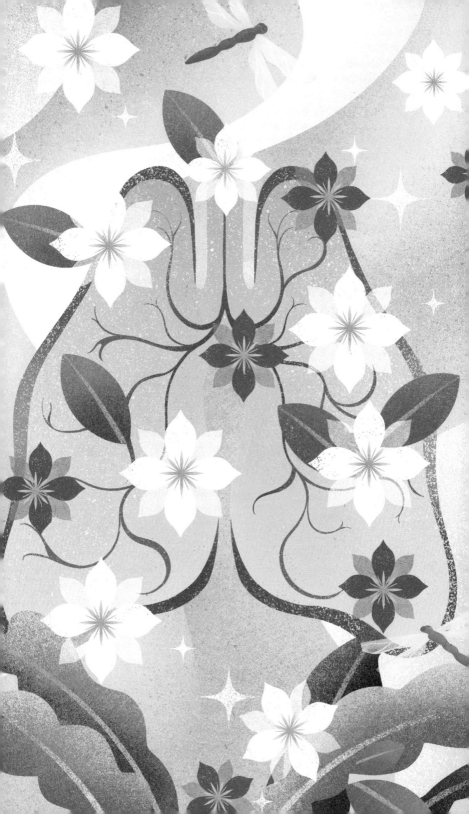

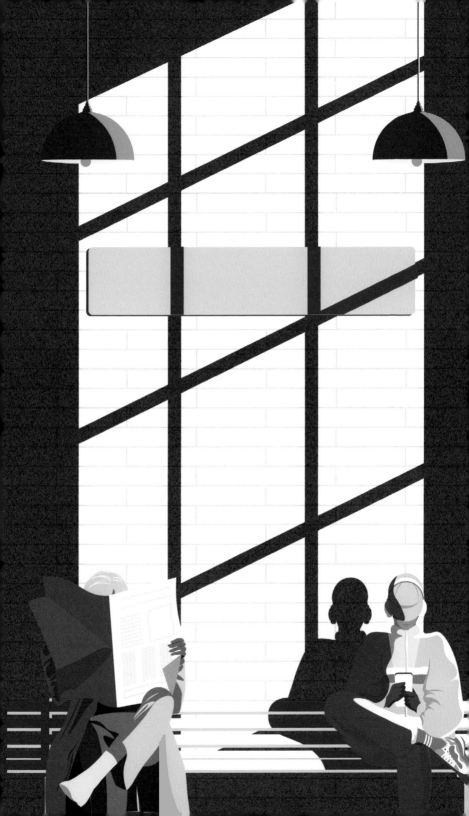

Bridging the divide

How understanding the influence of brain development over a person's lifetime can help with cross-generational communication

Every generation feels misunderstood by the one before. It's a rite of passage, a fact of life. This gap can result in a lack of communication, strained relationships and a shared sense of frustration. Why is it sometimes so hard to make meaningful connections with people who are younger or older than you? According to Simone de Hoogh, founder of non-profit venture PowerWood, which works with neurodivergent young people and their families, there are two main reasons: brain development and hormones. These two factors and one other – environment – make a significant impact on how you feel, act and communicate. Understand how these interrelate through the various stages of a person's existence and you might just make a breakthrough when it comes to communicating with those at a different point in their life from you.

Life-stage differences

Of course, not everyone feels that it's hard work talking to an older relative or worries about how they're perceived by a younger contact. Many empowering and mutually respectful relationships are formed across the generations, enhancing friendships in a wonderful way. But it's also common to simply not know what to say or how to say it, which can make conversations feel stilted and awkward.

Simone explains: 'We all live in our own reality and these differ depending on our culture, background and personal circumstances. It can therefore be challenging for the different generations to understand each other's habits and views on what is "normal".'

She goes on to describe how this plays out in a situation that is common in society today: 'It also explains why some of the older generation, who grew up playing on their own in the woods and fields without any computer access, find it difficult when exposed to, say, the fact that children aren't often given the freedom to play outside unsupervised, spending many hours online instead.'

But with a little research and a determination to be more understanding, it's entirely possible to reverse these feelings. And it all starts with how your brain processes information and how that changes as you age, from the very beginning of life to the very end.

Developing brains

The most significant stage of brain development starts while a baby is still in the womb, just three weeks after conception, according to a 2018 paper by neuroscientists Robbin Gibb and Anna Kovalchuk. Over the next two years, the brain changes and grows at an amazing pace, mastering everything from fine motor skills to language and facial recognition. Of course, not all children develop in exactly the same way, but every brain is still remarkable.

As we age, these great leaps might not be so noticeable, but 'our brains never completely stop changing, so that we rightly say that brain development starts shortly after gestation and ends with death', write biopsychologist Sebastian Ocklenburg and neuroscientist Onur Güntürkün in their book, *The Lateralized Brain*. In general terms, as you get older, changes include a shrinking in the frontal lobe and hippocampus, and declining synaptic connections. This might result in more frequent lapses of memory or finding it harder to learn something new. But it's important to remember that ageing is not uniform and cognitive abilities remain unique to each person.

Teenage years

Teenagers, too, undergo a significant shift, experiencing an intense period of change as their brains begin to mature and develop. While the brain grows into understanding the consequences of an action, teenagers are often characterised as reckless with their words and behaviour. That doesn't mean communication is impossible, but it may require a little more thought.

Simone says: 'Understanding brain development and hormone changes helps us to communicate more effectively because we can recognise why we or the teenager behave the way we/they do. Knowing that it's because of these changes allows for more empathy towards ourselves and our children. It facilitates us to see through the surface problem towards compassion for the young person and how they are feeling in the world.'

The same also rings true for those older than you. Taking time to remember the environment in which older generations grew up is helpful. Understanding how they feel in the world and avoiding age-related stereotypes is also vital. Your brain never stops changing and many people remain curious and open to learning throughout their lives. Entering a conversation with no preconceptions is a challenge, but one that ultimately pays off when you learn that you have more in common than you initially thought possible.

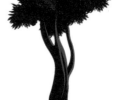

Power of empathy

Understanding each other better and letting go of age-related stereotypes has a positive knock-on effect on society as a whole. But if you find yourself continuing to struggle with difficult communication, Simone believes it's time to start looking inwards to see where the issue might be: 'I have used the knowledge about brain development to re-parent myself, mostly by learning to show myself a lot of compassion and calm down my own nervous system, with help of the awareness mantra and the 4-7-8 breathing exercise [see panel, overleaf]. This way I am able to relate to my children from a place of calm rather than from the stress that I experience when in a cycle of emotional and sensory overload.

'Over the years, I've discovered that my brain was stuck in juvenile ways of thinking, coloured by the trauma in my childhood. New knowledge and tools have led me to be more understanding of myself and my children. Patience and self-forgiveness when I slip up has helped me form new neural pathways more suited for a grown-up (and a parent), and shows my children to be compassionate with themselves as well.'

Through the ages

Applying compassion to yourself, forgiving yourself when you slip up and understanding why you feel the way you do can help influence your communication all the way along the spectrum of ages. Your positive behaviour can form the framework for a member of the younger generation to model themselves on. You can also employ that empathy to better understand someone a generation or two above you.

Communication expert Faith Valente, a professor at Gonzaga University, Washington in the US, agrees, and says that empathy not only helps increase understanding, but is also an important 'personal characteristic that facilitates our ability to persuade others to accept an idea, feel a particular way or pursue a certain course of action'. She goes on to say: 'Empathy is a communication tool we use every day to understand others and to share our thoughts, feelings and personal experience.' Naturally, not everyone will communicate in the same way, and that might not have anything to do with age. Simone, who herself identifies as neurodivergent, knows how hard it can be for people to feel understood when they don't fit into so-called normal patterns of behaviour and interactions.

A curious mindset

Communicating across the ages is a challenge that most people will face at various points in their life, but it's not something to dread. Engaging a mind that's curious about how the other person feels and the context of their life, and working hard on empathic communication will smooth the path towards fulfilling and fascinating conversations. There's so much to be gained and so little to be lost when you take the time to listen to someone, whether that's a teenager or an older person – life is made up of these shared experiences.

EXERCISE YOUR EMPATHY

Use the following two exercises to help calm your nervous system and show yourself compassion.

Awareness mantra

This is a simple tool you can apply every time you become aware of an unhelpful thought or memory, to prevent it from triggering subsequent unhelpful involuntary behaviour. Say the following to yourself (if possible, out loud):

I'm proud and grateful to be aware that I have/had a not-helpful thought/flashback/sound/picture/film/smell/feeling/action.

- Choose the most appropriate word based on the type of memory or action.

- Every time you become aware of an unhelpful thought, feeling or sensation you can apply the mantra.

- For instance, after feeling overwhelmed by an argument, you might become snappy. As soon as you're aware, you can say: 'I'm proud and grateful to be aware that I have an unhelpful feeling (being overwhelmed) and action (the snappiness).'

Follow this up with the 4-7-8 breathing technique.

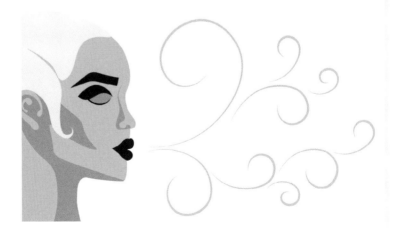

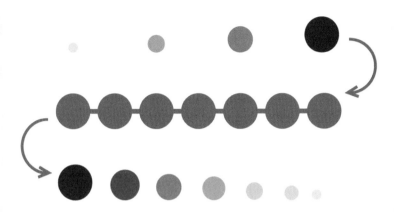

4-7-8 breathing technique

- Before you begin, place the tip of your tongue on the roof of your mouth just above your teeth, and keep it there throughout the exercise.

- Exhale completely through your mouth quite forcefully, so you make a 'whoosh' sound.

- Close your mouth and inhale quietly and softly through your nose for a mental count of four.

- Hold your breath and count to seven.

- Next, exhale completely through your mouth, making another whoosh sound for eight seconds in one large breath.

- Now inhale again and repeat the cycle three times.

Remember: all inhaling breaths must be quiet and through your nose, and all exhaling breaths must be loud and through your mouth.

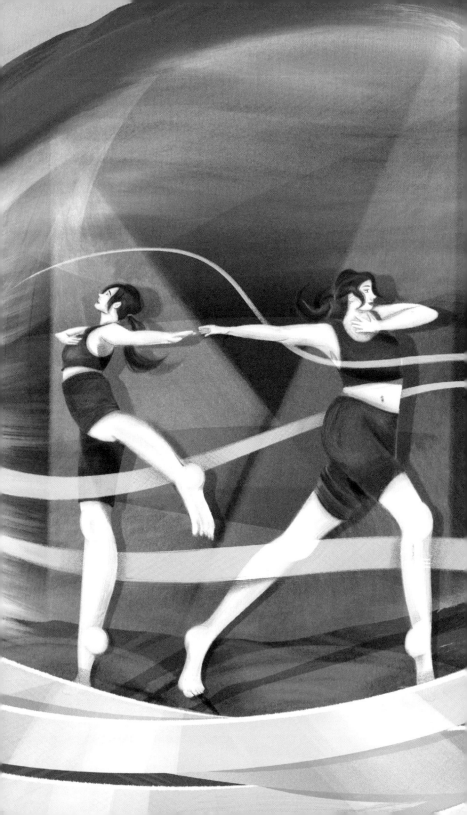

On body and soul

How to nurture your mind-body-spirit connection

Have you ever caught a glimpse of your reflection and noticed the difficult emotion you'd been struggling with written all over your face? So much of what goes on in your body is a mystery. In the same vein, you might have started a yoga practice only to discover a profound tightness you had no idea was there, or pain and tension you'd been holding in your body without being aware of it.

The truth is, many people spend vast amounts of time lost in thought, worrying about the future or ruminating on a story from their past. But what if we paid more attention to what's going on inside ourselves in the here and now – and the way our thoughts and feelings were being played out in our bodies? It sounds obvious, but it's surprisingly easy to forget that everything begins and ends in the body – that is experiences, the things seen, the people interacted with, the emotions felt and the thoughts had.

Making a connection

Our body is our means to being in the world – and it's the reason we literally carry around the difficult experiences we've had. To use an expression often quoted in relation to the body-oriented therapy Somatic Experiencing, 'the issue is in our tissues'. It's no wonder, then, that we view our physical self as the sum of who we are. Yet this is only part of the picture. Because, while every body is a manifestation of the physical and emotional experiences it's had – from the springy energy of a young child to the slumped shoulders of someone experiencing depression – this is only one aspect of what it means to be human.

Ultimately, our physical bodies offer a gateway to our inner life, the truest part of us, according to author and spiritual teacher Eckhart Tolle, where the 'joy of being emanates'. He believes many people are detached from the essence of who they are, a state of being he calls 'inner spaciousness', which goes beyond mind or personality. Eckhart writes of the formless self that transcends the body after death as both who you really are and the energy field of your body. But how do you reach this part of yourself? The first step is by learning how to be present in your body, and acknowledging the physical impact that your emotions have on you. Everyone has a window of tolerance, but life can push you out of your range of optimal functioning. To thrive, you need to learn how to put yourself back together again. If you don't, and instead avoid difficult feelings and physical sensations, you can increase the chance of feeling overwhelmed by them.

Somatic stress

In *Burnout: The Secret to Unlocking the Stress Cycle*, researchers Emily and Amelia Nagoski examine what happens in the body when the limbic system – known as the emotional brain – is constantly activated and gets stuck in the fight, flight or freeze mode. They break this down into a series of steps that begin with a stressor, an event or situation that occurs in the external world, such as sitting in heavy traffic on the way to work every day or constantly having to be polite to a difficult colleague. This turns into stress – the physical symptoms felt in the body, such as an increased heart rate, tense shoulders and shallow breathing, and can lead to more pervasive symptoms such as sleep disturbances and digestive issues.

The crucial part, they say, involves giving the body the resources it needs to complete the stress cycles that get activated every day. This could include any physical activity you enjoy, such as walking, running or swimming, or even just tensing all of your muscles before releasing them while sitting at your desk.

'Remember, your body has no idea what "filing your taxes" or "resolving an interpersonal conflict" means,' they write. 'Speak its language, [which] is body language.' But what happens when you don't manage to complete the stress cycle and those difficult experiences and feelings stay with you?

Unearthing past traumas

According to somatic movement specialist and yoga therapist Aimée Tañón, by fostering a strong mind-body connection, you can learn how to be more resilient when difficult, and often deeply held, feelings arise.

'The fact is there's a strong link between difficult physical sensations and difficult emotions or feelings,' she explains. 'During my classes, we'll go into a pose and it might feel tense – there may be some stiffness or mild pain there – and this often triggers the memory of a story or difficult event from the past. That's because these events are actually buried deep in our tissues.'

The important thing, Aimée asserts, is to learn how to feel this, to stay with it and then let it go. 'When we learn to breathe through the discomfort and feel the sensation of our muscles releasing, we develop self-knowledge and become empathetic with ourselves.'

Taking a step back

Taking this form of interior knowledge or intelligence further, psychiatrist Bessel van der Kolk describes the process of interoception as an 'awareness of our subtle sensory, body-based feelings'.

Rather than completing the daily stress cycle or meeting difficult sensations on the yoga mat, interoception is a process that enables an individual to stay calm and take control before a stressor can make an impact by learning to take a more objective view of the situation. In doing so, it's possible to override the emotional brain, instead activating the medial prefrontal cortex, the part of the brain responsible for choice-making.

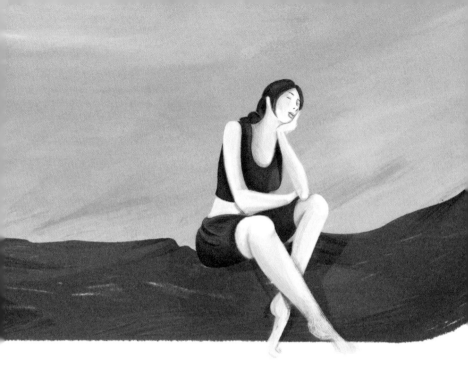

Giving emotions form

It's no surprise then, that one of the best ways to cultivate interoception is through a mindfulness practice. In a recent talk on the fear of ageing and loss, meditation teacher, psychologist and author Tara Brach describes a state of bodily awareness that transcends stressors by going to the heart of difficult emotions, and feeling their shape, texture and even temperature.

'When we worry about what's ahead, how our body is going to change – whether we're afraid of turning 30 because we fear a decline in physical attractiveness or an increase in responsibility, or we're afraid of turning 75 and fear losing control of ourselves and becoming more dependent on others, we tighten our bodies,' she says. Notice the way anxiety feels in your body, and how you're being pulled into a story, by anchoring yourself in the present moment, she says. 'Pause for a moment and ask, what is this situation trying to teach me?'

Showing up

Of course, it can take courage to do this, especially as paying attention is the opposite of distraction – an operating mode that can be at play in many people's lives. But it's something that, according to Buddhist nun, author and speaker Pema Chödrön, we're more likely to achieve if we can learn to come from a place of kindness and self-acceptance, and engage in a process that calls us to be present. Tara agrees: 'Only then can we develop intimacy with our inner life and each other. Only then can we connect to our inner beings – that transcend our bodies – and remember our belonging to spirit.'

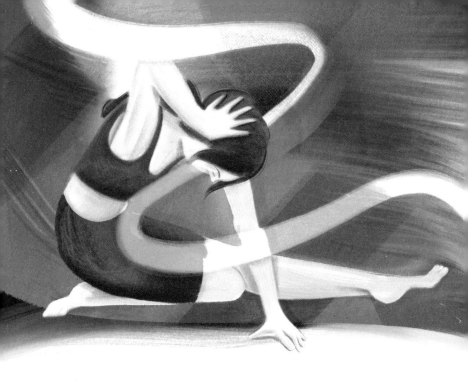

HOW TO FOSTER A STRONG MIND-BODY-SPIRIT CONNECTION

Ground

According to holistic health therapist Kate Edwards, noticing how your body makes contact with a surface, in a practice known as grounding, is a great way to foster bodily awareness.

- Find a comfortable position, either sitting upright in a chair or on the floor.

- Notice the sensation of your feet making contact with the earth, pressing down through the heel. Or the feeling of your legs on the floor where you're sitting.

- Feel that sensation of being held – in your seat or by the ground, feeling supported.

- Now notice your breathing, and the feeling of your muscles.

- Notice any places that feel more relaxed, or neutral.

- Focus on the softness and expansiveness in your body.

Greet

While practising grounding, you might start to notice tension in the body accompanied by difficult thoughts and feelings.

- Try to meet the edge of that emotion and soften – allowing yourself to feel vulnerable. Greet any difficult emotions and give them form by jotting them down here.

....

....

....

....

....

....

....

....

....

....

....

....

....

- Feel the knot and the heat, the 'daggered' feeling in your chest. Allow yourself to sit with it until it's no longer uncomfortable. At first you're allowing the feeling – and then you're making friends with it.

- As you lovingly release difficult emotions, this is when you might feel the heart breaking open. It's possible you'll reach a vast tender space, a place of belonging.

Complete

Journalling can be one of the best ways to 'drop into the body' and complete a grounding and greeting practice.

Start by describing how you're feeling in this moment. Remember you are writing for yourself, so use the pen to record any combination of words or images that come to mind – however unusual they may seem.

....

....

....

....

....

....

....

Next, try to focus on your body. Are there any tight areas still? Make a note of them here.

....

....

....

....

....

....

....

....

Where did you feel pain in the grounding practice? You might come up with descriptive words, like hot, heavy, sticky or jagged, or an image.

....

....

....

....

....

If you managed to release that difficult emotion in the practice, how did it feel? Again, allow any descriptions or images to come to mind.

....

....

....

....

....

Finally ask your body a question: is there anything else I need to do to complete this practice? Note the answer you get without judging or altering it in any way.

....

....

....

....

....

'The best of life is conversation'

Ralph Waldo Emerson

Reaching out

How talking to strangers in a safe space could enlighten your day

Most children are given strict instructions never to talk to strangers, to keep them safe. Many adults spend part of their day surrounded by strangers, yet the idea of striking up a conversation with someone they don't know often feels uncomfortable. In cities, being openly friendly to someone unknown can be seen as socially unacceptable, or even odd. The mere thought of it can for some be intimidating and anxiety-provoking, so self-imposed isolation remains the norm.

Mood-booster

But not everyone sees it this way. Judy Apps, a TEDx speaker and author of five popular books on communication, likes to consider the positive effects that a spontaneous chat with someone you don't know could have on daily life. 'There are amazing possibilities [that can] come from a conversation with a stranger,' she says. 'These interactions can be life-affirming and energising, for both parties. Even a 30-second conversation can lift your mood.'

It can be easy to underestimate what connecting with others in this way can do for your own and others' wellbeing. Conversely, many people overestimate the level of discomfort they'd feel if they were to reach out to a stranger. 'We're all different, some are naturally chatty and others aren't. Some are more introverted and not used to putting themselves out there,' says Judy. 'I think it's about not being too hard on yourself.'

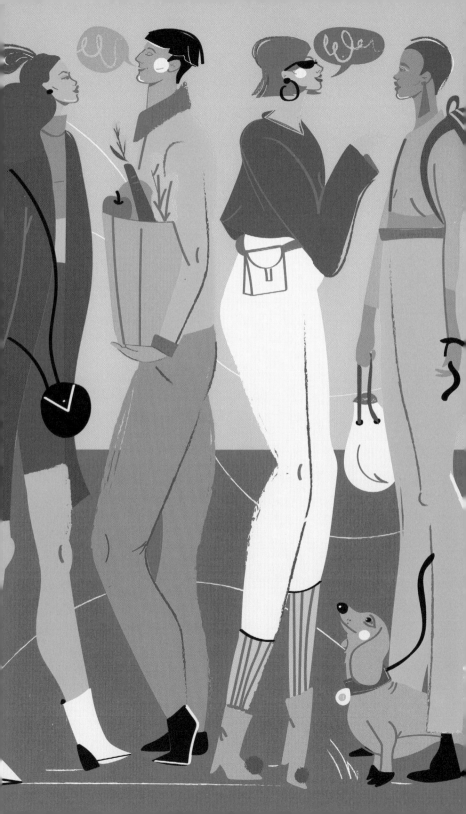

Good together

Are the potential benefits worth taking the leap into the unknown? There's a growing body of research that suggests engaging with and trusting people you don't know is important for personal and communal wellbeing as well as the health of society. Friendly behaviour to strangers has been linked to higher self-esteem in teenagers in the US, while in China, greater trust in strangers has been linked to better overall health.

Studies suggest people might be short-changing their own happiness by ignoring opportunities to connect and talk to people around them. 'It's amazing how something that feels like a genuine exchange can warm you and make you feel you're not on your own on this Earth,' says Judy. 'The impact is much greater than realised. Saying something can easily make somebody's day. It's like seeing a rainbow – you're so thrilled by it that it carries you through into the next few hours.'

Effortless exchanges

Judy sees the art of conversation as being like a game of bat and ball. 'You both reveal a bit about yourself at each back and forth,' she says. 'You quite quickly know whether you're connecting as people or not.' This year, BPP University Law School, which has an online campus plus centres in London, Leeds, Hong Kong and Berlin, launched what's thought to be the world's first module in small talk, created after internal polls found 43 per cent of students feared strangers would judge them according to how they spoke. The aim of the module is to arm students with skills in chit-chat and networking to build real connections after graduation.

What's holding you back?

If we're to get started on our own, it's important to identify existing roadblocks between ourselves and a great conversation with someone unexpected. An increasing reliance on tech could be one of them: a recent study found that phones can keep people from even exchanging brief smiles with people they meet in public.

It's also important to know your audience. In Finland, for example, people feel that if there's no important topic to discuss, there's no conversation worth having. One of their national sayings is: 'Silence is gold, talking is silver.' Meanwhile trying to start a chat with the person sitting next to you on the plane at the start of a six-hour flight might not be welcomed. 'Where people can't run away, a bit of silence can be great,' says Judy.

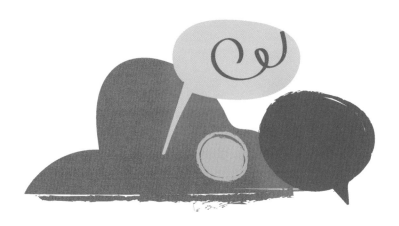

Nothing personal

Being mindful of your surroundings when approaching a potential exchange with someone new is important, and so is keeping things light. 'It's often said the best way to start a conversation is to ask an open-ended question, but I don't think that's true,' she says. 'Try floating a non-threatening comment without heavy expectations and just see what happens. If you get no response, nothing is lost. Nine times out of 10 you'll get something back, even if it's just a friendly grunt. The smallest response can seem great if you've not spoken to anyone all day.'

The UK might be better at this than imagined. 'In England, people are always talking about the weather,' she says. 'We toss a statement out into the ether like "Wow, sunny today isn't it?" to see what happens. It's nothing personal and that's what is important. The other person can catch hold of it if they want to. If the interchange is warm and friendly, there's an added feel-good factor for both parties.'

Wonders for wellbeing

And for people living on their own, such face-to-face interactions, however fleeting, can be important for wellbeing. Humans are social creatures, and feeling isolated and lonely can pose a health risk that is comparable to smoking or obesity. If you're feeling shy, taking a light-hearted approach can help. 'The next time you pop into a local shop, say to yourself: "I'm going to say something." By setting this goal and making it into a game you can throw out a sentence. Even if no one responds you can give yourself brownie points for trying.' However, it's one thing to strike up an exchange, but another to make it more meaningful, says Judy. 'Meeting anybody and discussing the weather is nice. But if you feel somebody has understood you in a brief conversation, which often happens with strangers, that can really touch your heart.'

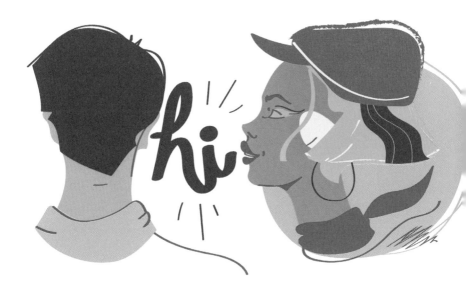

Fresh eyes

This is something Adrià Ballester, founder of the Free Conversations Movement, wants people to experience, just like he did for the first time in 2017. After a particularly bad day at work he decided to go for a walk through his native Barcelona, instead of bringing home negative energy. 'I happened to get talking to an elderly man, we talked about everything and anything and I came away feeling so much better, calmer and with a new perspective on my own situation,' he says.

The next day he started up his movement, with the aim of creating spaces where people can freely express themselves. He picked a spot, set up two chairs and a sign saying 'Free conversations', and waited. 'What's really interesting is when someone sits down you have no idea what they'll say or even what language they will speak,' says Adrià. 'Whenever we start a conversation with a stranger we should be open to whatever the other person is about to tell us.'

Inside help

He has only two ground rules: he will not judge and he never gives advice. 'I've learned that most people are happy to talk, and even a short exchange will do a lot of good. I see people really connecting with themselves in the moment and I've never had anyone check their phone while we've been talking, which is nice.' He adds: 'I believe some conversations can save lives and that's why I started this movement.' With the help of a band of volunteers, Free Conversations has extended its reach to Warsaw, Dublin and Lisbon, and has a strong global online following. 'I've got to talk to people from all over the world with totally different points of view to mine,' says Adrià. 'The experience has helped me open up and adopt a new perspective, which is beautiful.'

GET TALKING

Follow these five tips for starting a conversation with a new person in a safe and personally fulfilling way.

1. Bat and ball

Most exchanges start with a mundane subject, like the weather. To move it on, throw out a non-threatening comment. If you receive a positive response, be a little braver next time and tag a question on the end. All being well, the chit-chat should go back and forth, like a game of bat and ball.

Conversation starters to try...

- Lovely day, isn't it?
- It looks like it's going to rain.
- I hear there's going to be thunderstorms all weekend.
- Can you believe this weather?
- Doing anything fun at the weekend?
- I can't believe how busy/quiet it is today.
- What's your dog's name?
- You look like you've got your hands full.
- How long have you been waiting?

2. Rise to the challenge

If you find it difficult to talk to people, set a goal for next time you go into a populated area. When the opportunity arises, make a little comment. The response is not the result, the result is that you did it. Give yourself a high five for talking to someone new.

Use the space below to note down what you said and the response you received. These can serve as positive reminders next time you need a confidence boost.

....

....

....

....

....

....

3. Believe in the magic

It's amazing how quickly and easily an exchange with a stranger can become a satisfying conversation if you're willing to be vulnerable for a minute and open to what might happen. Something beautiful can take place in a real-life exchange with little effort.

4. Read the room

The moment you start talking to somebody, look for affirmations, not just in the words they're using, but in their tone of voice or whether their face lights up when they speak. Ask yourself: 'Does their body language match what they're saying?'

Positive signs:
- Leaning in shows real interest.
- Feet pointed towards you signals engagement.
- Touching an arm indicates trust.

Signs that you may want to change the topic:
- Shoulders raised to the ears indicates embarrassment.
- Rapid blinking can be a sign of anxiety.

5. Get the balance right

Of course, there are times when you'll need to protect your personal safety. If a stranger seems hugely interested in you and is overly flattering, or you feel they're trying to get closer to you but aren't giving anything away about themselves, be cautious. These can be warning signs for you to stay on guard. Look for a sense of equality and balance in any new interactions and trust your instincts – they can be your best allies in such situations.

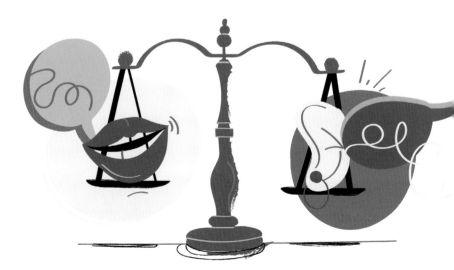

Use the space below to document conversations that worked well and those that didn't, as something to refer to back to. If you like, make a note of any thoughts that were going through your mind at the time alongside.

Forward thinking

A kind act not only benefits someone else, it can be good for you, too – so pass it on

'When you get, give. When you learn, teach.'

Maya Angelou, the acclaimed author and civil rights activist, believed that this advice, passed down by her mother, was one of the greatest lessons she'd ever learned. It could also describe the concept of paying it forward, where a physical item, knowledge or a kind or positive deed is passed from one person to another. It demonstrates that you don't have to be rich or powerful to have a positive impact. After all, you can set a pay-it-forward chain in motion just by smiling at a fellow shopper or commuter. Uplifted by the experience, they too might extend your friendly greeting to another passerby and, before you know it (in fact, you won't know it), your goodwill could have radiated out into the world in the most wonderful way.

Ancient concept
The idea, of course, isn't new. It can be traced back to ancient Greece and has been practised through the ages by great thinkers. There are also modern-day examples, including Elizabeth Nyamayaro, whose memoir, *I Am a Girl from Africa*, was published in April 2021. As a child in Zimbabwe, Elizabeth was rescued from starvation by a UN worker, whose actions made such an indelible impression on her that she was inspired to devote her life to humanitarianism.

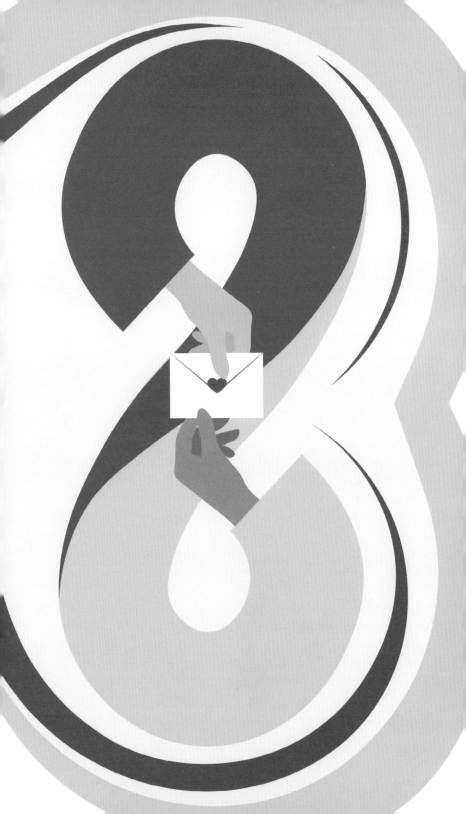

Contagious and spontaneous

There are everyday moments of kindness, too. One morning, in the winter of 2012, a woman at a drive-through coffee shop in Winnipeg, Canada, paid the bill for the customer in the car behind her. The recipient of this generous act then chose to pay it forward, too, setting off a ripple effect of altruism that continued, with each of the subsequent 228 patrons paying for the car behind them.

Other examples include coffee donations for rough sleepers, meals for those who need them, free commercial flights for people seeking to do good in the world and even pay-it-forward programmes for organ donations. This happens at Loyola Medical Center, near Chicago in the US, which runs an altruistic kidney-donor scheme.

Perhaps one of the best-known examples came in 2006, when broadcaster Oprah Winfrey handed out $1,000 debit cards to 300 studio audience members, inviting them to experience what she called 'truly the best gift' of giving. The results were heartwarming. One woman took a group of young people, who might not otherwise have had the opportunity, to see *The Nutcracker* ballet. Another audience member used the money to kick-start a project to transform a barren courtyard at a veterans' medical centre in Seattle. In the end, Oprah's kindness warriors gave out gift cards, paid for petrol and groceries for others, supported victims of domestic abuse, and donated to hospitals.

Importantly, each of these people did more than take time out to ensure the money went to fantastic causes. Their generosity inspired companies and communities to get in on the act, and a snowball of kindness rolled across the US, with many of those involved describing the joy and satisfaction these seemingly selfless acts brought them.

Sense of reward

The scope of these acts is also wide. Studies have found that simply witnessing a generous deed can inspire generosity, allowing a single moment of kindness to spread goodwill to others. Research also suggests that doing good deeds increases a person's wellbeing. It can give a sense of purpose, boost self-esteem and increase feelings of gratitude and compassion. In turn, nurturing these emotions can have a positive effect on health by helping to reduce stress and anxiety. In short, kindness has a lot going for it, and passing it on seems to have even more.

TIPS FOR PASSING ON GOOD DEEDS

- Generosity is meant to feel good, so it's important to give only what you can afford.

- Be creative and vary your kind deeds and gestures to keep it fun and prevent them from becoming a chore.

- Look out for opportunities and be prepared to extend your help to strangers.

- Pay attention to when others' gestures and behaviour benefit your life, say thank you and consider emulating them.

- Giving doesn't need to be about money. Often, the most valuable gifts are time, knowledge and skills, which don't need to be big or showy.

- Don't wait for someone else to start a chain of goodwill, set the domino effect in motion yourself.

- Give without expecting anything in return. If someone does offer to repay you, suggest they pay it forward.

- Consider volunteering for a group or organisation and enjoy the camaraderie of being part of a kindness team.

Paying it forward can start with the simplest gesture. Perhaps the first could be to consider what small act of kindness you could set in motion today?

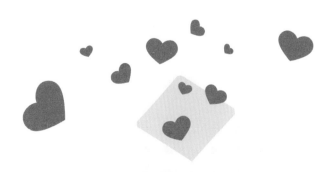

NEED INSPIRATION?

Here are a few ideas:

- Offer to mentor someone in your field of expertise or teach someone a skill you have.

- Spread good news and uplifting stories.

- Bake for your colleagues, neighbours or friends.

- Call or visit a friend, relative, neighbour or an older person who might be isolated.

- Buy from a small, local business.

- Pass on a book you've really enjoyed.

- Leave positive little notes in library books or paint uplifting messages on stones and leave them around your neighbourhood for people to find.

- Make new people feel welcome in the places you know well.

- Pay for the person behind you in the queue.

- Donate unneeded clothes, furniture and so on to charity.

- Offer to babysit the children of parents who don't get out much.

- Be forgiving when someone makes a mistake.

- Take on pro-bono work if you can afford to.

- Donate to a local food bank.

- Send an impromptu handwritten letter or card to someone you know.

START TODAY

Paying it forward can begin with the simplest gesture. Use this space to explore small and inexpensive moments of kindness and the difference they could make to people's lives.

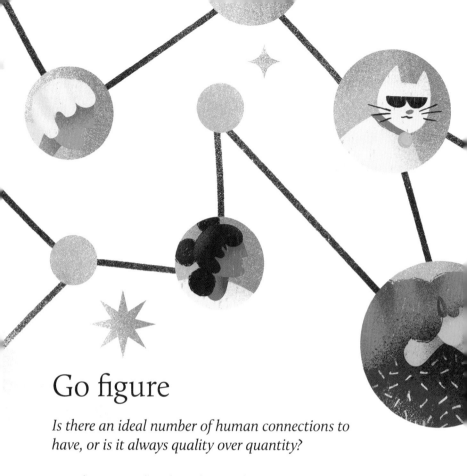

Go figure

Is there an ideal number of human connections to have, or is it always quality over quantity?

According to British anthropologist Robin Dunbar, 150 is the magic number. He believes that this figure is the maximum amount of stable social relationships a person can handle. But it's just part of the wider story when you're counting the number of people you know.

Social genetics

Dunbar suggests that 150 is the maximum number of people in your network with whom you can be expected to maintain relationships. More than that and you move into acquaintance territory, which can become unstable. Fifty is the approximate size of a friendship circle, while 15 good friends is about right, and the number of very close friends, or loved ones, is five.

But what does this say about human bonding? To ascertain the numbers, Dunbar explored correlations between the size of non-human primates' brains (specifically their neural networks) and the size of their social groups, through neuroimaging and observing time spent on grooming and other interactions. He concluded that the size of the brain, relative to the body, was linked to social group size. He then applied this formula to humans, discovered that historical and anthropological data supported it – and 'Dunbar's Number' was born.

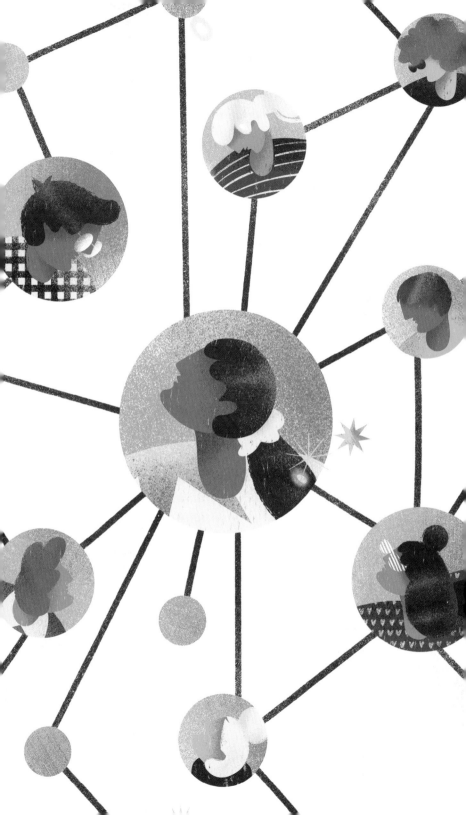

Keeping in touch

This theory came into existence during the late 1990s and much has changed in the way humans communicate and socialise since then, not least the rapid and ongoing expansion of social media. The average number of friends a person has on Facebook varies between 130 and 330, while for a personal Instagram account, it hovers between 100 and 200. So, why accrue so many 'friends' on a platform where you might only engage meaningfully with a handful? Coach and neuro-linguistic programming practitioner Rebecca Lockwood believes the answer might be a reflection of how we feel about relationships in real life: 'We can sometimes get caught up in how many friends we have if we're feeling lonely or if our relationships are not very strong,' she says. 'I try not to think about the number of friends I have, but I do think a lot about the quality of my relationships and making sure I stay in touch with people. I always have dates in the diary for catching up with friends and make it a habit to get another date booked in before we part. It's important to remember that if someone hasn't responded to a message, it's nothing personal, it's just that life has passed by. I always follow up with people.'

Real encounters

The lines become more blurred when you use social media to promote your business as well as to update your network on your private life. Rebecca believes a firm divide can help keep the two separate, but also recommends taking a step back when the desire to start comparing yourself to friends and acquaintances creeps in: 'If social media ever becomes overwhelming or you find yourself feeling negative after using it, this is a good indication that you need to take a break from the platforms and check in with yourself. Take the time to connect with friends in real life. Social media can be a brilliant tool for keeping in touch with people and staying up to date with what they have going on, but if it ever begins to feel negative, then you can try to change this by changing the way you relate to it.'

And this might well be the key to making use of Dunbar's Number. Any time you feel overwhelmed by the scale of casual acquaintances you've amassed, taking a step back to reconnect with close, real-life friends can be the remedy.

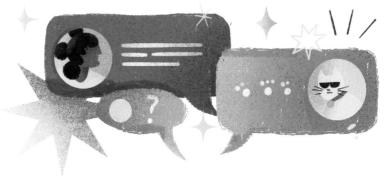

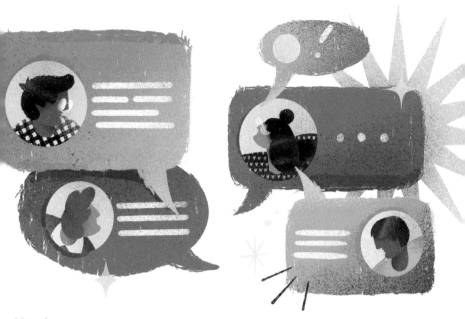

Meaning matters

Whether online or offline, having a group of close friends is still important and has many physical as well as mental benefits. US science journalist Lydia Denworth says: 'The most important finding in the science of friendship is that people (and animals) with better social relationships are healthier and live longer. In humans, social isolation is as much a risk factor for health as smoking.'

And the quality of those relationships is just as important, more important, in fact, than the quantity. Watching those numbers creep up on your social media channels or knowing lots of faces when you're out and about provides a momentary lift. It's one that appeals to the ego, but ultimately does little to soothe the soul.

Natural selection

But is there any benefit to cutting out those in your online and real-world circles who bring little to your life in the form of genuine connection? It's a tough decision to make and one that can have repercussions. But the chance to free up time to understand the relationships that mean the most to you can bring a greater awareness of where your priorities lie.

Rebecca has experienced this herself: 'The dynamic of my relationships with friends I was once really close to changed when I had my children. My relationship with my younger sisters also changed, as they don't have children and we stopped being interested in doing the same things. I no longer wanted to go out drinking or to do the things they wanted to do. It's not always easy in these situations and it's normal to mourn the loss of strong relationships, but we also have to be mindful that we grow and move through life at different rates, and sometimes change the outlook we have and the things we're interested in as a result.'

Put yourself first

Friendships can and do change. Friends come and go. Maintaining numbers for the sake of it runs the risk of being counterproductive. Chasing an ever-increasing figure could tear you away from that core two or 10 who really matter to you. Perhaps it's the pull of something new that draws you towards adding to your network. Or maybe you're ready to move on from old relationships but haven't plucked up the courage to leave them behind. However you manage your circle of friends and acquaintances, it can be helpful to ask yourself the following question, being as honest as you can with your answer:

Is there a limit on the number of people in your life you can meaningfully engage with, and how does that affect your relationships with those closest to you – your core friendships?

Ultimately, numbers are just that – numbers. What matters most is you. And we're all different. Those who gain confidence and energy from being in a large group of people might tend to have larger networks, whereas those who prefer more intimate connections will appreciate perhaps one or two close friends. Everyone else will fall somewhere between the two. It's an old adage, but quality over quantity couldn't be truer when it comes to relationships. Hold those closest to you closer and don't feel bad about stepping away from less meaningful connections.

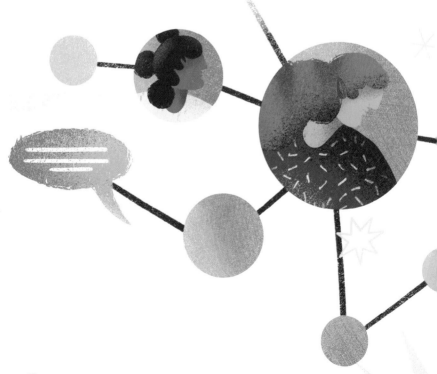

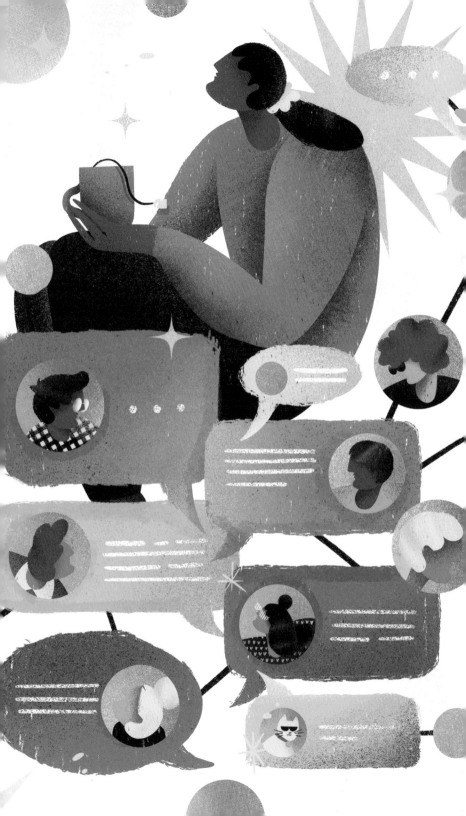

SKETCH YOUR CIRCLE

- Taking a blank piece of paper, start by drawing a small circle. Inside, write down the names of those who form your closest relationships. Ideally, list no more than five.

- Draw a larger circle around this one and inside write down the names of your good friends. Try to keep to an upper limit of 15.

- After this, draw another circle around the second one. Thinking of your wider circle of friends, write down their names. This might include up to 50 people, but fewer is fine, too.

- Finally, draw a larger circle again and write down the name of those people you're in touch with regularly, but wouldn't class as good friends. Aim for no more than 150.

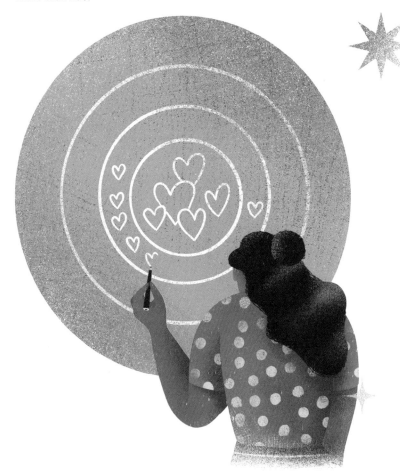

You could use your sketch to help you to see your relationships more clearly. Think about who you didn't include on the list. What does this mean to you?

....

....

....

....

....

....

Are there names that you might like to move towards the centre, or others you feel belong further out?

....

....

....

....

....

Are there any actions you could take to ease this process?

....

....

....

....

....

WAYS TO STRENGTHEN A FRIENDSHIP

- Be intentional with your time. Put an agreed date in the diary to meet up and on the day of your catch-up make sure the next date is agreed before you leave.

- Think of a time you shared that really made you laugh. Write a text, message or email to your friend to remind them of it.

- Remember the details. Mark a date in your diary that your friend might not remember – when you met, your first holiday together, a special picnic.

- Be vulnerable and trust them to support you. Even if you're not someone who feels comfortable sharing your inner thoughts, take a chance on a good friend and talk things through with them. You'll build trust together.

- It might not be their birthday, but a funny card or package through the post can lift someone's day.

- Make it about them. The art of conversation relies on you listening more than talking. Ask questions and really listen to the answers. If there's something ongoing that they're dealing with, remember to follow up on it next time you talk.

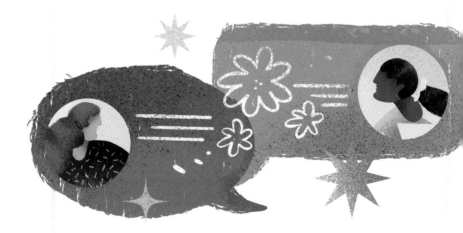

WORK TOGETHER

Working towards a shared goal can help form great connections.
Getting fitter, joining a book group – what might you both commit to?

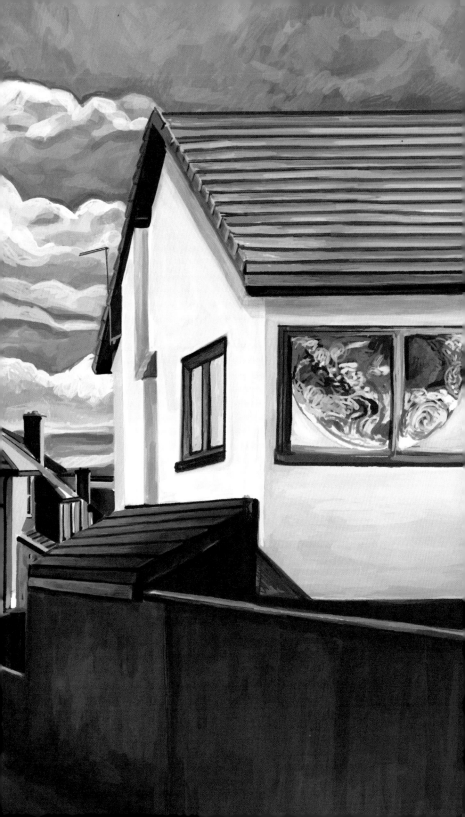

In a small world

*How living with fewer distractions can create room for
big things to happen*

Recent global events forced the majority of us to close our doors to the outside
world. We had to shrink the spaces we occupied. We could no longer stretch out
our limbs and spread ourselves so widely. The world became smaller, but did that
mean we minimised ourselves with it? Or did the world, along with ourselves,
become more potent? With fewer distractions, did you become more present?
Perhaps it allowed you to see things that had always been there, but which you'd
never quite noticed...

Paring back

For me, this hunkering down was already a deliberate choice. A couple of years
ago, I swapped the city for the countryside and a lower-key, less complicated life.
A smaller, and therefore simpler life, would mean there would be fewer decisions
to be made. And for an indecisive person like me, that prospect was heavenly, as
with fewer things to choose from, the pie chart of my life wouldn't have so many
segments. I've never been good at maths, but it seemed to me that life's equations
were being simplified by going small.

Now, I have a greenhouse and vegetable boxes in the garden, I grow onions,
cauliflowers, potatoes, beetroot and garlic. The garden is mercurial, and some
changes are so slight that you'll only notice them if you pay close attention. Have
you ever seen a tomato plant grow from seed? The seeds are so tiny they'd get lost
if you held them in your hand and sneezed. Yet they push their way through the
soil, determined to feel warmth and light. They grow tall and strong and it's so
exciting to see them one day adorned with yellow flowers – soon to be tomatoes.
To witness transformations such as this requires patience.

Increased awareness

I never paid attention to life's nuances when my own was busier and full. When you become engrossed in something so wholeheartedly, whatever it might be, it becomes its own planet – a world to be inhabited in awe and wonder. You become not just a voyeur, but a participant.

This small-world absorption isn't only for those in rural areas. It can happen anywhere. A friend, who lives a busy and varied life in a city, says that since being at home more, she's noticed that a squirrel arrives in her garden at the same time every day. She laments the fact that she'd never noticed it before being asked to work and stay at home where possible, but has now gone out of her way to learn all about these acrobatic creatures. She's discovered that red squirrels are rarer than grey ones and that, apart from the obvious difference in colour, they're smaller in size and have distinctive, large ear tufts.

Though the pandemic forced many to make their physical horizons narrower, perhaps, in doing so, some lives have been expanded. My friend didn't have a clue about squirrels before. She's now more knowledgeable – her appreciation of life has been enhanced. The squirrels have always been there, but she hasn't always been present enough to enjoy them. Perhaps there's a case for living more deeply than broadly?

Same old, same old?

The German philosopher, Immanuel Kant, might be seen by many as a rather dull man. For 40 years he woke up at the same time every day – 5am. He would lecture at university for exactly four hours. He had lunch at the same restaurant at the same time every day. In the afternoon he would go for a walk, taking the same route through the same park at the same time. He never left his city. But he described space and time in such a way that it inspired Albert Einstein's discovery of relativity. He proposed the idea that animals should have rights, and he invented the philosophy of aesthetics and beauty. Kant's daily routine might seem limited and narrow, but who would argue that his achievements weren't huge?

'The secret of happiness, you see, is not found in seeking more, but in developing the capacity to enjoy less'

rates

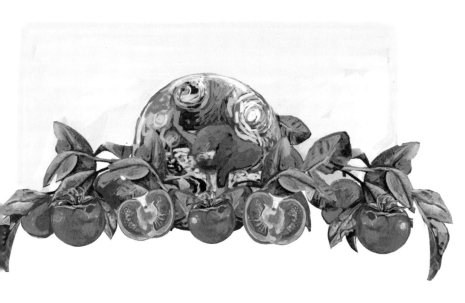

Honing in

In fact, there are many examples of people who have chosen to eliminate choice in their lives in order to focus their mind on things that really mattered to them. Returning to Einstein, the physicist wore variations of the same grey suit every day because he didn't want to waste brain power worrying about clothes.

It was the same for personal-computing pioneer and Apple co-founder Steve Jobs. His attire? Blue jeans, black polo neck and trainers. Even Socrates, credited as one of the founders of western philosophy, is said to have walked barefoot around the markets in Athens, happily declaring how little he needed in order to be content. Choice is so often presented as desirable – to be 'spoilt for choice' is deemed a plus point – but maybe it's an unnecessary distraction, a complete time-waster even.

Less is more

Perhaps it's a misconception that we need endless variety in order to find adventure and meaning. Some of the greatest minds have not lived broadly, but deeply. They chose the worlds they wished to occupy and lived inside them. Everything outside these areas was superfluous. Eliminating choice, and therefore living small, allowed them the space to become experts in their fields and influence worldwide thinking. It illustrates how living small can have a big impact, as well as the benefits of zooming in on your interests and choosing a life that some might call microscopic, but that has purpose.

Everyone is free to choose the world in which they exist. What I thought was living small has given me a bigger experience in life. I have narrowed my focus, expanded my knowledge and engaged more fully with my surroundings. I don't regret my old life, it's just another way of being. But I'm grateful for a different perspective. Bigger is not always better.

LOVE YOUR SCALE OF LIFE

- Focus on what you have and enjoy what you're doing, however simple those pursuits might seem. Don't be dismissive about the smaller pleasures in life. It's not always about the big experience.

- Immerse yourself in the things you enjoy. Read about them, study the ins and outs – expand your knowledge and your world.

- Think carefully about the choices you make and their value to you and to the greater scheme of things. Distinguish between want and need.

- Take time to think about all your accomplishments, including those that seem less significant. Congratulate yourself for having done them.

- Revel in the process of nature. Whether this is planting seeds on a windowsill or planning a new pollinator-friendly garden border, nature teaches patience and the importance of nurture.

- Understand that you are free to occupy the worlds that you choose – whether that's woodturning and baking or philosophy and Jane Austen novels. The choice is yours and yours alone.

- Know that just because you've scaled down, it doesn't mean that your life is less full or impactful. It's quite the contrary, in fact, because your life is full of the things that you have chosen.

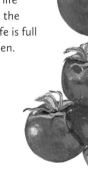

MY ME-TIME LIST

Think about crafts or subjects you previously enjoyed that have fallen by the wayside, and list them here. Why might this have happened? If it turns out there just didn't seem to be enough hours in the day, how can you make time for them?

....

....

....

....

....

....

....

....

....

....

....

....

....

....

....

....

....

....

Tender is the life

How a combination of courage, curiosity and compassion could lead to a softer-hearted world where everyone benefits

The moment my dad first scooped my newborn daughter into his giant hands, cupping her head and body the way he must have done when I was born... The stranger who asked if I was okay when I started crying in a cafe... The first time I saw the glittering arc of the Milky Way making its way across the enormous navy-blue night sky in Botswana... When I think about tenderness, these are some life events that spring to mind. In simple terms, tenderness is the capacity to be tender – sensitive to your own needs, those of others and the world around you. Because while the emotions behind these moments differ, what they have in common is an experience of being present with others and the way that lives are interconnected.

No time to stop
It goes without saying that this way of being can have profound benefits for you and the environment in which you live. It requires thinking from the heart rather than the head. And no matter who you are or what your life's been like, there will be moments of tenderness that weave through your days, ones you've created and ones created for you. It's possible for most people to live from a place of tenderness, approaching life with presence, empathy and kindness. Yet in a fast-paced world it can be hard to stop and chat to a homeless person, pause to notice the flowers growing between the pavement cracks or savour fully the food you're eating with each bite. It can even be hard to show up in this way for those closest to you – to show empathy rather than frustration when your partner has too much going on to support you or when a child is sick on the day of an important meeting. But why?

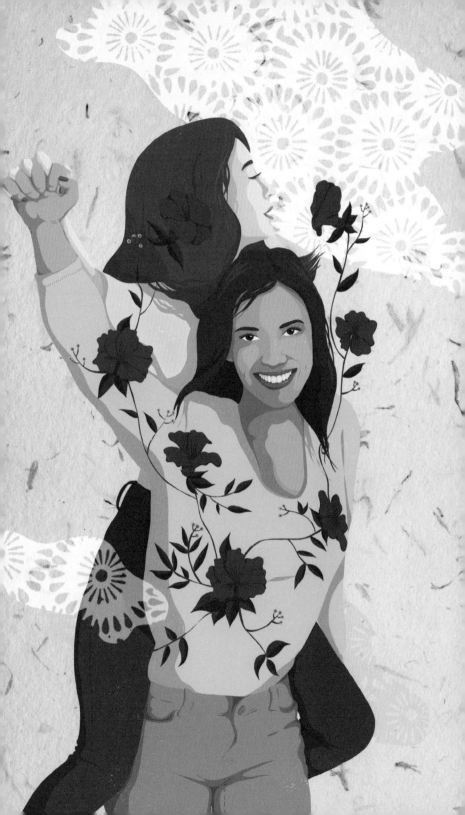

Keeping your distance

It can stem from a tendency to distance yourself from your emotional responses, pulling away from the people and events in your world rather than meeting life with your whole being. There are times when it can seem easier to ignore your true feelings and instead spend time overworking, staring at screens, or turning to alcohol or caffeine.

According to meditation teacher and author Tara Brach, this can happen as a result of patterns set during childhood, where caregivers who struggle with the unpredictability of life strive to control their environment by grasping and clinging to particular outcomes, constantly afraid of what might happen if they don't. This habit, however, is then passed on.

'There's this sense of wanting to control life and a feeling of threat if we can't,' she says. 'We feel it's our fault when things don't work out, and we interpret our environment as threatening and perceive others as a threat, even when there is nothing to be afraid of.'

Prioritising care

These overwhelming feelings are housed in the limbic system, which regulates much of what the body does and bridges the gap between the physical and psychological. When the limbic system is regulated, we're better able to manage our emotions. According to Manchester-based CBT therapist Somia Zaman, however, when you exist in a state of fight or flight and the limbic system – the emotional part of the brain that houses the amygdala and hippocampus – goes into overdrive, you switch from being open and receptive to the world to a heightened state known as shutdown.

'When this happens you're in basic survival mode and your brain is telling you that giving and receiving love and tenderness isn't a priority,' she explains. 'But kindness and compassion are really important in terms of survival because humans are social beings and depend upon "strokes", either physical or psychological, to feel good.' The irony, however, is that when you're finding things difficult, the default position is often to blame yourself. 'Learning how to be kinder to yourself and accept the kindness of others is extremely important,' adds Somia, who says experiences of compassion can form a protective barrier against mental health problems.

Path to tenderness

So how do you come back to yourself, to the tenderness that lies deep within your heart, the soft spot that's the core of most people? The first step is by accessing courage to act differently towards pain when it surfaces, to notice it and sit with it, rather than ignoring or masking it with distractions.

These responses are wired into the neural pathways, however, and it takes conviction and determination to make a change and approach things differently. Courage is needed to pause because that's when it's possible to begin to notice what's going on. As a space opens up, it's then easier to become aware of thoughts and begin to question their ultimate truth – and to wonder if they're having a harmful effect on your state of mind.

The next stage involves adopting a curious mindset. Asking questions about yourself, others and your environment can encourage more empathy and a sense of embodiment in the world. Living from a place of curiosity means being aware of a new way of being, seeing things outside yourself rather than remaining stuck in a negative internal thought loop.

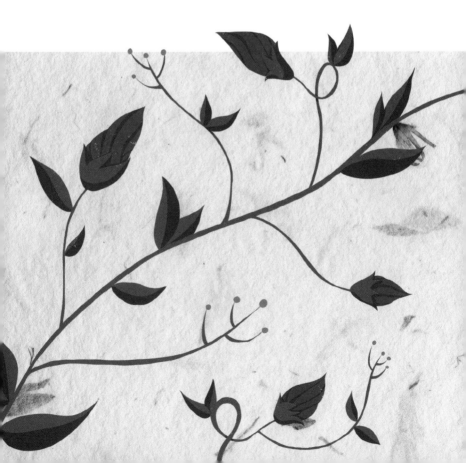

Natural empathy

Finally, start to reach for compassion. This is born out of a deep-wired desire to care – for yourself and others – that is underpinned by kindness and benevolence rather than duty or fear. It's something Dacher Keltner, professor of psychology at University of California, Berkeley, aims to prove through his work at the Greater Good Science Center. He says the evolutionary argument that humans are instinctively self-serving – greedy, selfish and motivated by money, fame and power – is inaccurate. As evidence, he refers to Charles Darwin's assertion in *The Expression of the Emotion in Man and Animals* that the most successful communities are those with the greatest sympathy for their members. They have the most offspring and provide them with the best care, proving that the drive is rooted in human biology and that there's an evolutionary basis to compassion. In fact, the act of compassion, giving a warm smile or a friendly wave, releases oxytocin – the hormone responsible for making us feel more kindness – into the bloodstream.

Physiological impact

Compassion shows up in the brain as well as the body. According to one study at the University of California, for example, brain imaging revealed that when someone witnessed another person in pain, the exact same area of the brain lit up as when they experienced physical pain themselves. This suggests that compassion – to care, feel for others and be part of a community – forms part of the structure of human DNA. But other instincts pull in different directions, so while a person might want to focus on love and care, they could also desire a thriving career. Similarly, someone might wish to be surrounded by chaos and adventure but also hope to find stillness and peace. Being human is complicated.

That's why it's important to remember that the ability to give has a limited lifespan without self-compassion. In fact, any extended period of giving without taking time to replenish the self can be draining. To give and receive is to become more present with others and to see how lives are interconnected. Who knows, it might even start a tenderness revolution.

'If your compassion does not include yourself, it is incomplete'

Jack Kornfield

CULTIVATE TENDERNESS IN YOUR LIFE WITH THE THREE Cs

Courage

A simple practice like box-breathing for a minute or two every morning can help you find space between the things that happen in your life – situations, people or events – and the way you respond to them.

- Start by visualising a box or square.

- Imagine drawing a line along one side of the box as you breathe in through your nose while slowly counting to four.

- Continue along the next side of the box as you hold your breath for four seconds.

- Draw the third line as you breathe out through the nose for four.

- Finally, create the last line as you hold again for four.

- Repeat the sequence five times.

- Now, jot down any challenging events or situations and explore your feelings about them.

....

....

....

....

....

....

....

....

Engaging in these practices daily can help you to find more resilience and reduce the impact of fear on your life.

Curiosity

One of the best ways to invite tenderness into your life is by adopting a curious mindset. You can do this by asking yourself questions. Try answering the following:

Why am I struggling with this feeling or situation?

....

....

....

....

....

....

....

What would it feel like to be another person and have to cope with their life?

....

....

....

....

....

....

....

At the same time, remember you have your own struggles and find life difficult at times. When you notice yourself becoming frustrated and making assumptions, take a moment to engage in a quick question-and-answer session, such as the one below. The answers could change your perspective and evoke empathy.

What is life asking of me?

....

....

....

....

....

....

....

....

Which is worse: failing or never trying?

....

....

....

....

....

....

....

....

When I'm in pain – physical or emotional – the kindest thing I can do for myself is...

....

....

....

....

....

....

....

Think of a compassionate way you've supported a friend recently. Now write down how you can do the same for yourself.

....

....

....

....

....

....

....

....

....

....

Compassion

Calling to mind people in your life and consciously appreciating them by seeing their innate goodness can help you to cultivate feelings of tenderness. Engaging in a short daily practice such as the one below can be a good habit to establish.

- Begin by sitting quietly and thinking of someone you find easy to love (this could also be a pet).

- See the kindness and capacity for love that flows through their being and imagine yourself offering them a gesture of care. It could be putting a hand on their shoulder or gently stroking their cheek.

- Bring to mind another person or being and see them when they're happy and expressing love.

- Again, imagine that gesture of care, and visualise communicating the goodness that you see, whispering words of kindness in their ear.

This practice is about seeing the field of love that's ever present, but to which it can often be hard to connect.

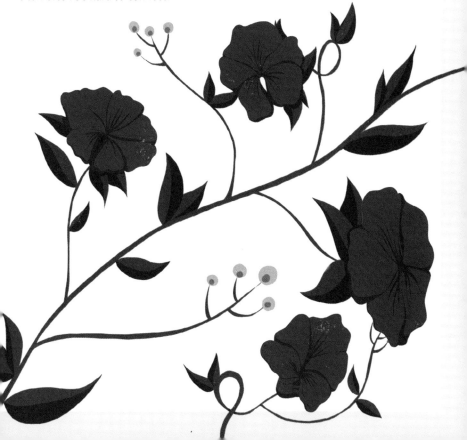

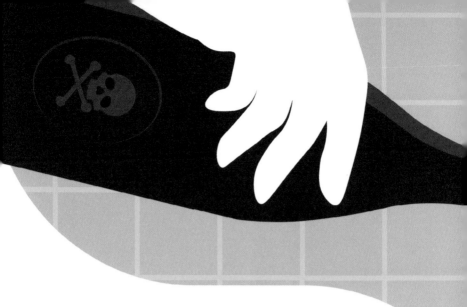

Out of harm's way

Toxic relationships can inflict a heavy toll all-round, but there are ways to help a loved one break free and find their true direction

By the time Chelsea* accepted that she'd been in a toxic marriage for 20 years, she felt that it was time to do something, but also too late to do anything at all: 'There were always red flags, right from the beginning, but you overlook them after a while,' she says. Chelsea met her husband Peter* through a mutual friend. After a couple of years dating, they broke up. She said the differences between them were too great, and she moved on. A few years later, Chelsea's sister ran into Peter, who asked her to say hello to his former partner and suggested she might call him some time. This led to hours of turmoil for Chelsea's sister as she debated whether to forward the message. Finally, she passed it on, while hoping nothing would come of it. Soon, however, the pair were dating again. Peter, it seemed, was a changed man.

Caught in the middle

At the time, Chelsea was living with her parents and helping to care for her poorly grandmother. In the wake of her grandmother's death, Peter revealed that he was going to be evicted and needed a place to stay. The obvious solution seemed to be for him to stay at Chelsea's parents', but they disapproved of unmarried people cohabiting. Chelsea recalls how the combined forces of not wanting to 'leave Peter stranded' or to upset her family 'pushed me towards marrying Peter'. The exchange of marital vows, however, led to far more than Peter's presence in the family home. It became a cycle of toxicity, from which, years later, Chelsea is still trying to extricate herself.

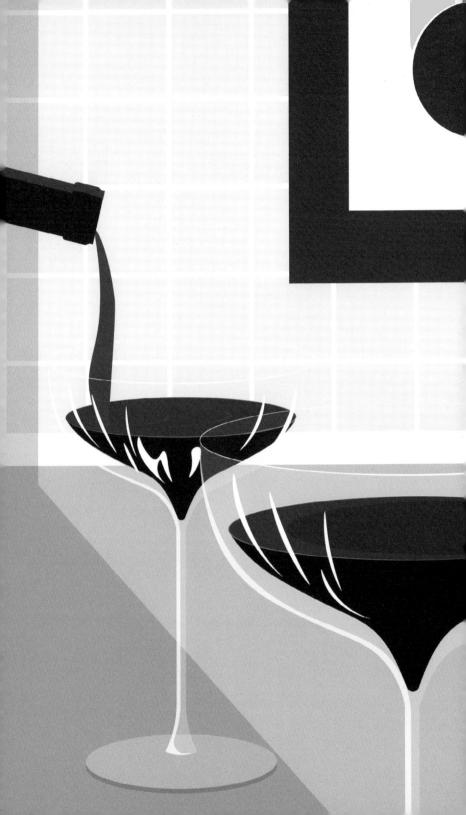

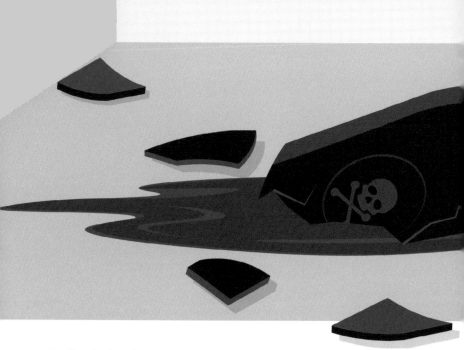

Feeling isolated

The truth was that while Peter was indeed a changed man, it wasn't necessarily for the better. In addition, secrets emerged about his earlier life that Chelsea felt compelled to keep hidden. These periodically resurface and cause great pain. Feeling forced to keep these struggles from her family, Chelsea's mental and physical health has been affected and she's become reclusive. Now, however, she's hoping to find the strength to move forward without her husband and reduce the anguish and chaos in her life.

Consequences of trauma and toxic choices

Professor Rose Marie Alonso-Chatterton, a licensed mental-health counsellor, believes people who find themselves in toxic liaisons have often experienced an earlier emotional trauma. 'Sometimes, they just don't realise what they've been going through until years later,' she says. 'Yet in many toxic situations, after a period of time, a person eventually loses their sense of self.'

For some, including Chelsea, the traumatic events become the only thing on which they can focus: 'Once you're in a toxic relationship, particularly one that's emotional and as intimate as marriage, your self-esteem is so intensely impacted in negative ways, you lose the ability to dream a different life for yourself,' she says. Sticking to a daily routine has helped her to survive the challenges of her marriage without having to address them. Rose Marie describes the attraction to toxicity as 'blind spots' – whether that involves things, behaviours or people that qualify as dysfunctional. They happen because of what a person 'has been exposed to in their lives over a period of time'.

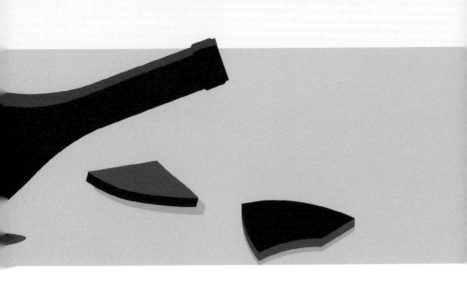

Right and wrong

In many cases, as in Chelsea's, it's harder to see the negatives when a relationship has shifted from positive experiences earlier on. When they were first dating, Peter was the life and soul of the party, he was sociable with strangers, took Chelsea to places she felt would be disapproved of by her parents and showed her a good time. 'He was so tough and brave. I felt like we could go anywhere together and I'd be safe, so I saw a lot and did a lot, too,' she recalls. And although they're constantly at odds, Chelsea says Peter is 'a great protector' of her mother. Rose Marie suggests that this is the moment when people begin to 'rationalise the things that are wrong, because they're deep into a relationship that feels both wrong and good at the same time'. At this point, their needs become secondary, and 'they begin to shift away from the things that are most important to them, like family, friends, personal interests and education'.

Witness to the scene

Throughout all of this, however, there's been another person whose life has been affected by Chelsea and Peter's unhealthy marriage, and that's Chelsea's younger sister. She blames herself for putting the pair back in touch and thinks that if only she hadn't passed on Peter's message then her sister's life would have taken a different path. There will be other well-meaning people who, intentionally or not, introduced a loved one to a seemingly charming person who turned out to be destructive.

Paying witness to such events takes a heavy toll, and knowing how or when to intervene can be challenging, complicated and dangerous. Rose Marie suggests trying to take steps as early as possible, and says there are several ways to try to break through the toxicity and help a loved one get where they want to be. It can't be achieved overnight, but change is possible. And so is self-forgiveness. So, while you're looking out for a friend or loved one, remember to be kind to yourself, too.

WAYS TO HELP

If you're concerned that a loved one might be in a toxic relationship, here are five things to bear in mind:

1. Dialogue
Talk to your family member about your concerns for them, without being accusatory or confrontational.

2. Active listening
The more you listen to your loved one about their situation, the more you'll understand what they're going through and what their needs are.

3. Boundaries
Keep a healthy border between yourself and your loved one's partner.

4. Contact
Offer invitations to activities, social gatherings or other interesting events that might help your loved one meet different people.

5. Support
Be available for conversation and identify changes in your loved one that might require action, legal support or a safe haven.

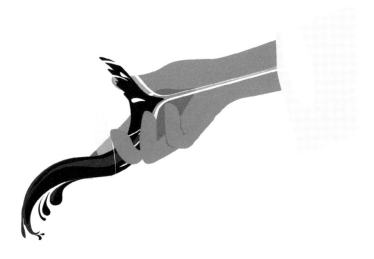

HOW TO FIND A PATH OUT

Here are some prompts to work through for anyone in a toxic relationship:

A first positive move is a change in mindset. Understanding and believing that a toxic relationship must end is central to breaking a vicious cycle. Get your thoughts down on paper so that you can view them more clearly.

....

....

....

....

....

....

....

....

Reclaim a sense of self and personal identity as early as you can and in a way that makes sense for your lifestyle. In other words, begin to think for yourself about who you are. When do you feel happy? When have you felt the most happiness in the past?

....

....

....

....

....

....

....

Start small. Show yourself you can try something different, just for you. This could include starting a course, learning a new language or trying a new hobby outside of your household responsibilities. What activities could you try?

....

....

....

....

....

....

....

Confront the shame of what's happened in the relationship. Understand that it's not your shame, and it's been put upon you. This is a personal conversation to have with yourself. It does not involve confronting your partner. Be as honest as you can.

....

....

....

....

....

....

....

....

NEXT STEPS

When it feels comfortable or safe to do so:

- Tell your family you're making changes to your life and they must immediately desist from having any contact with your partner.

- Meet new people when possible and discover where your interests lie.

- Join a support group. Talking to people who share and understand your experience will open up conversation and opportunities for change.

- Consider talking to a therapist or counsellor. One-on-one dialogue can help to discover how best to approach a situation.

- Change your own dialogue about the relationship.

- Make no excuses for bad, unwelcome or negative behaviour towards you by your partner.

- Work out a plan and find a safe passage to leave the relationship for good.

- Share what's happening with someone you trust implicitly. If you have no one, try calling a confidential helpline.

For more information, and to find helplines for men and women, visit the Mental Health Foundation at mentalhealth.org.uk (search for 'toxic relationships').

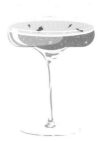

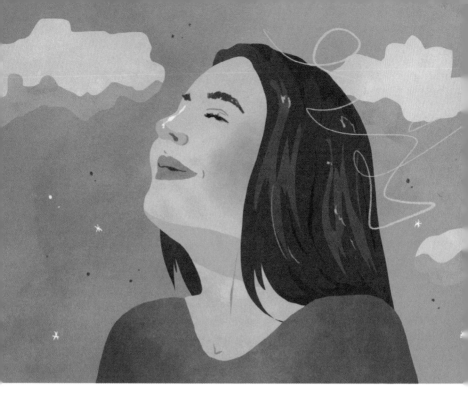

More than words

A lot has been said and written about the positive power of affirmations, yet many struggle to harness their benefit. Here's how to tailor and channel these phrases in ways that serve your needs directly, linking to desires you'd like to manifest

The observation by Gautama Buddha that 'We are what we think' rings strikingly true for those who've experienced this phenomenon through the practice of mindfulness, hypnotherapy or similar exercises for the mind. Dwelling on beneficial ideas through the use of affirmations is another way to overcome patterns you might like to change. In addition, affirmations are believed to lower stress levels, decrease anxiety and improve focus, concentration and confidence.

If you've used them before, have you done so successfully? Perhaps you've seen some improvements, or maybe you started off with constructive intentions but gave up when you didn't notice a big enough shift? If that's the case, you're not alone. There are various factors that can impact their effectiveness. However, armed with more knowledge, you might be surprised at the difference a few adjustments can make.

Power of words and intention

The wording you choose for your affirmations is important, and how and when you use them can affect their success. Change often occurs on a subconscious level, so it's crucial to employ the kind of language to which your subconscious is more likely to respond. Fortunately, there are techniques that can help to establish successful affirmations, and strategies that can increase the likelihood of a positive outcome. Here, we explore a few of them and suggest a way to create your own guided visualisation process.

While nurturing a desire to realise your affirmation is key, cultivating a deeply felt intention is also fundamental to its success. Before you start using your affirmations, check in with yourself to feel your intention. Try to feel it in your body, like a gut instinct. Is it a sense of excitement or determination? Or something else? What place is it coming from? What are your reasons and motives for wanting to manifest it?

You can enrich your intention, strengthening and moulding it. How much do you want this? When you have a sure sense of the feeling, focus on encouraging it. Remember to keep your intention strong yet relaxed, deep but effortless. It's important for it to be firm but surrounded by a gentle energy, like the arts of tai chi or qigong, where less is more. Keep the sense of your intention with you at all times. To do this, you might like to imagine your intention as a precious shell, a crystal or a lotus flower – something you nurture and feel connected to.

Wonder of relaxation

Affirmations are most effective when you're relaxed, which is when the mind is more open to change. One way to make the most of this state is to practise some self-hypnosis techniques. This might sound tricky, but self-hypnosis is just a term for changing your mindset during a relaxed state. You can enter natural states of hypnosis over the course of your day. Like hypnosis, self-hypnosis is about passing on helpful messages to your subconscious. The subconscious mind likes to please, so if you can connect with it, you can tap into many possibilities.

You might also like to jot down your affirmations overleaf, then try 10 minutes of mindfulness or play a guided relaxation session of your choice. Once you're in a relaxed state, drop in your affirmation, repeating it 10 times or more. Spend another few moments in this relaxed state, then repeat your affirmation again. Set an alarm to go off after 15 to 20 minutes if you think you might nod off. Try not to work with too many affirmations at once. If you have two or three that are linked to the same theme, that's fine, otherwise stick with one for each self-hypnosis session. Practise self-hypnosis once a day for a week, review your progress and continue for longer, if need be.

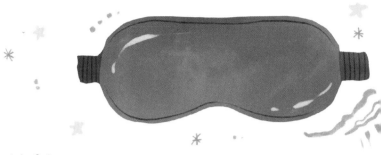

Potential of sleep states

You can use affirmations at any time during the day, but before bedtime is effective. As you drift into sleep, try mentally reciting your affirmation. This pre-sleep phase is called hypnagogia, and is similar to a hypnotic state, so if you apply a suggestion or affirmation at this point, you might find it has a hypnotic effect.

Another effective time for employing affirmations is when you're waking up in the morning, which is also regarded as a phase when you're in a type of hypnotic state. Before you're fully awake and out of bed, try to lie still with your eyes closed and recite your affirmations. They can also be combined with some self-hypnosis, as your mind will already be fairly relaxed.

Creative visualisation

Another way of manifesting and strengthening affirmations is through creative visualisation, which focuses on an end point to bring you results. A visualisation mobilises the brain and body's natural resources and is a powerful way to help manifest change. Repetition is part of it, so try to repeat your visualisation regularly. You might like to record something that is tailored to your specific goals, needs and dreams.

Learning styles

In broad terms, learning styles can be categorised into three types: visual, auditory and kinaesthetic. About two-thirds of the population are said to be predominantly visual learners. If that sounds like you, you might find visualisation exercises fairly easy. If not, use a mode that suits you.

If you're mostly an auditory learner, where music, talking and sounds resonate, try reciting a story or playing a piece of music to expand or forge a link to your affirmations. On the other hand, if you're a kinaesthetic or tactile learner, you will like to feel the change you want to make. To encourage a real sense of what it would be like – physically, mentally and emotionally – to achieve your desires, tap into what that would feel like to touch or smell. You might even like to use a pebble or crystal to hold while you're reciting your affirmation.

Hypnotherapy or self-hypnosis isn't recommended if you have psychosis or certain types of personality disorder. If you have any concerns, see your GP before attempting any self-hypnosis exercises.

HOW TO CREATE SUCCESSFUL AFFIRMATIONS

1. Use the power of now
When writing affirmations, it's more effective to use the present tense and first-person narrative, as if the experience is already happening – for example: 'I feel calm during the busy mornings.'

2. Be positive
Avoid negative words, including 'don't', 'no', 'doesn't' and 'not'. The subconscious responds far better to friendly and positively framed instructions.

3. Tailor your affirmation to your situation
If you're struggling with the amount of sleep you're getting, you might try: 'I sleep deeply and wake feeling refreshed.'

4. Put it in your own words
Your subconscious will respond better to your personal language quirks, rather than unfamiliar ones.

5. Have a strong intention
Motivation and intent play an important part in the success of affirmations. Try to cultivate a deep inner belief that what you'd like to happen will happen.

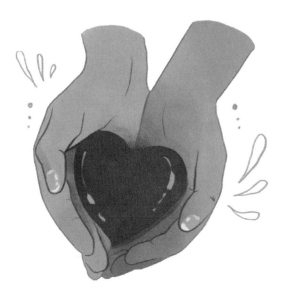

CREATING YOUR OWN GUIDED VISUALISATION

You might like to prepare a self-guided visualisation by writing and recording your own script. It can help to start by including ways to relax your body – we've included a body-scan meditation here to get you started:

Mindful body scan
This meditative exercise connects mind and body. Make yourself comfortable in a room where you won't be disturbed. Lie on your back on a mat on the floor, or on your bed. Legs can be flat or knees raised, whichever is most comfortable. You might wish to rest your head on a cushion. Now, you're ready to begin:

- Allow your eyes to close and take a few moments to get in touch with the sensations of your body, listen to your breathing and feel your back and limbs making contact with the floor or bed. On every out-breath, allow yourself to let go, slowly sinking a little deeper into the mat or bed.

- Starting with your head, focus on feeling its weight as it rests on the cushion. Now introduce your forehead, noticing if there is stress or tension. Then include your eyes, nose, cheeks, mouth, chin and, finally, the ears. What sounds can you hear? Be aware of the changing sensations in your body and the pattern of your breathing. It's natural for thoughts to wander, so don't worry if this happens. Just guide your mind back to your body.

- Slowly, shift your focus to the areas where the shoulders are in contact with the floor or the bed. Notice the strength in the muscles here and whether they're holding tension. Breathe into any tightness and let it go on the out-breath, releasing it from your body. Extend your awareness into your arms, elbows, wrists, hands and fingers.

- With care, bring the focus to your chest. Tune in to the subtle rise and fall with each in- and out-breath. Think of the ribcage and your upper back resting on the floor. If you notice any tension, aches or pains in these areas, breathe into them and out again, releasing them from your body.

- Bring your focus gently to your legs. Feel their weight, from the tops of the thighs to the bottom of the ankles. Notice any sensations. How are they resting on the floor? Is there numbness or tingling?

- Finally, move your attention to the feet. Allow the focus to follow all the way from the underside of the toes along the soles and around the heels. When ready, breathe in and feel the sensation of your breath as it moves down your body and into your toes. On the out-breath, feel it returning upwards, releasing any tension or discomfort. Repeat this pattern between three and five times.

- When comfortable, take one or two deeper breaths, before returning to your regular breathing pattern. Open your eyes and spend a few moments here before gently easing your body to a sitting position. Again, take a few breaths before standing, making sure you are comfortable and steady.

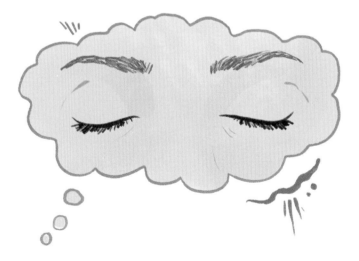

NOW CONTINUE YOUR SCRIPT...

Create a narrative around your goal and bring your affirmations to life. Describe what you might see if your affirmations came true, as well as what you might hear, smell and feel. Are you alone, or is someone with you? Weave in your affirmations, and any other desirable suggestions you'd like to work towards. Keep all wording in the present tense, as though your affirmations are currently taking place, such as: 'I speak with confidence and credibility.'

....

....

....

....

....

....

....

....

....

....

....

....

....

....

....

....

....

....

Read and record what you've written above slowly so that when you listen to your recording it follows a gentle pace. This allows images and messages to fully develop in your imagination.

When you're ready, find a quiet space, close your eyes and listen to your recording. Allow your imagination to go on a journey. Remember to pack your intention – this is the ace up your sleeve to realising your goals.

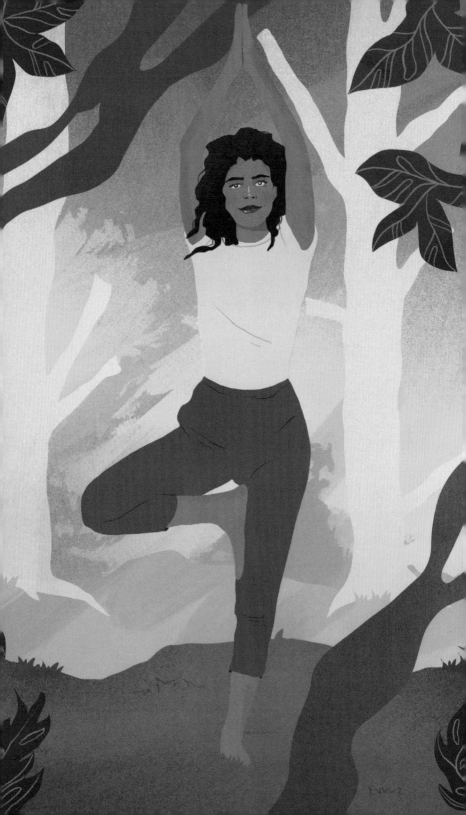

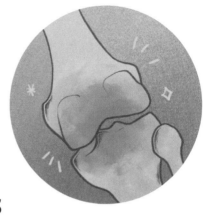

Happy hinges

Looking after your joints is an often-overlooked aspect of wellness, but it can have real and lasting benefits, so it helps to do what you can to keep these important connectors in good health

When Dorothy meets the Tin Man in *The Wizard of Oz*, he's been stuck for about a year holding his axe aloft, his joints stiff with rust. But a quick splash of oil on the elbows and knees and he's soon dancing happily along the yellow brick road. If only joint care in the real world were that simple.

While many people make their fitness and wellbeing a priority, joint health is often overlooked. In fact, some forms of exercise, such as road running, can do more harm than good if proper care isn't taken to protect the joints. And all the meditation in the world won't help you unwind if you're too stiff to sit on your yoga pillow.

A broad remit

Looking after your joints is a fundamental cornerstone of good health because it affects so many aspects of life. Focusing on better joint health can enhance your performance in your favourite sport or hobby, or simply your ability to walk upstairs. It can allow you to sit at your desk more comfortably or help you get a good night's sleep. It improves balance, range of movement and also offers a better chance of recovering after injuries and maintaining quality of life as the years roll by. You're never too young to start thinking about what you can do to boost your joint health, but it's also never too late to make improvements.

Complex structures

Joints function like the body's hinges, connecting the bones using complex systems of cartilage, tendons, ligaments and muscles. Depending on what's being defined as a joint, there are between 250 and 350 of them in the human body, including the ball and socket (like the hip or shoulder), which allows movements in all directions, and the hinge joint (such as the knee and elbow), which opens and closes in one direction. Wherever there is movement in the bones, from the jaw to the toes, there are joints involved. Because they are such complex structures, with different types of tissue working together, they are vulnerable to injury and disease, such as arthritis, which causes pain and inflammation. Osteoarthritis, sometimes known as wear-and-tear arthritis, is the most common form, and occurs when the cartilage is damaged over time.

New perspective

David Vaux, an osteopath and exercise lead for the charity Arthritis Action UK, says people often only start thinking about improving their joint health when they're in pain. If you're struggling to climb the stairs because your knees hurt or you can't sit at your desk to work because of a flare-up of back pain, then those crisis points might be the times when you seek medical help. Joint pain is extremely common and although there are specialists, such as osteopaths and physiotherapists, who can help in the short term, the long-term road to better joint health is one that you have to walk yourself by committing to certain lifestyle choices.

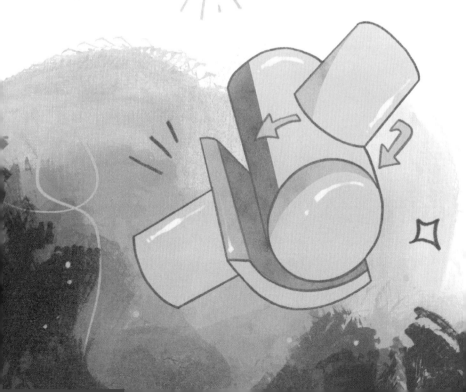

Let's get physical

David says the two most important changes you can make are to increase (or start) strength training and maintain a healthy body weight. He suggests that a well-rounded exercise plan includes strength or resistance training, plus flexibility sessions, such as yoga or Pilates. Luckily, the former doesn't have to mean lifting weights in a gym, either. There are plenty of body-weight exercises you can do in your own home, such as squats, push-ups, hip raises and lunges. Adding free weights, such as dumbbells, will increase the intensity, but do some research or seek professional advice as to how to use them safely. Resistance bands are also useful for home workouts.

'Ideally, people should be doing a minimum of two strength-training sessions every week from their teenage years onwards,' says David. 'Think about it as being strong for life. Being strong is the antidote to frailty.' David also explains how weight affects the joints. 'If you lose 1lb of body fat, that's the equivalent to a 4lb load across your knees when you're walking. So, if you lose 10lb then that's like putting down a 40lb rucksack.'

Leading the way

In Japan, there is a tradition of doing 10 minutes of exercise every day, which has been credited with maintaining mobility as people age. Japan's public broadcaster, NHK Radio, airs a show called Rajio Taiso – translated as radio calisthenics – early every morning. It features a series of musically led warm-up exercises suitable for most people. First broadcast in 1928, with the aim of improving public health in Japan, the show has become part of Japanese culture, with people gathering in parks and community spaces to move together as part of their morning routine. The first part of the Rajio Taiso programme focuses on improving fitness at any age – including exercises that can be done from a chair – and the second specifically targets improving strength.

Taking good care of your joints as part of your regular routine could be seen as 'pre-hab' – preparing yourself for the stresses that life will inevitably put on your body. David describes patients who have led active lifestyles still skiing and dancing in their 90s. 'You could think of yourself as an athlete and that the event you're training for is life,' says David. 'Looking after your joints at whatever age is an insurance policy for your independence in the future. Most people face illnesses and injuries at some point, but you can picture yourself as a fighter, training in advance to be able to withstand those blows that life throws at you.'

FIVE POINTERS FOR JOINT 'PRE-HAB'

1. Be strong for life
Aim for at least two simple strength- or resistance-training sessions each week (see overleaf). If you're new to strength training, there are plenty of online resources and videos to get you started and many exercises can be done at home (search 'strength exercises' at nhs.uk for a helpful starting point).

2. Mix it up
If you stick to the same exercise routine then your physical health might plateau. Try out new hobbies or classes, different online tutorials, or go rambling with friends. Keep challenging your body in different ways.

3. Consider a daily 10
If you're new to exercise or want to make it a more integral part of your day, take inspiration from the Japanese and try to move for 10 minutes every morning.

4. Try to maintain a healthy body weight
Remember that making even small changes can be beneficial for joints. If you think you might benefit from losing a significant amount of weight, seek advice from a health professional to do it safely and sensibly.

5. Tweak your diet
There are many joint supplements out there, but eating a wide variety of natural, unprocessed food and plenty of fruit and vegetables is helpful. Try to avoid refined sugar, trans fats and excessive alcohol consumption, which can increase inflammation.

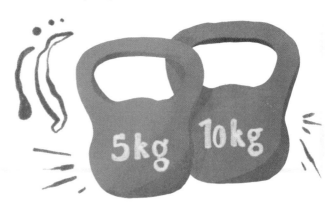

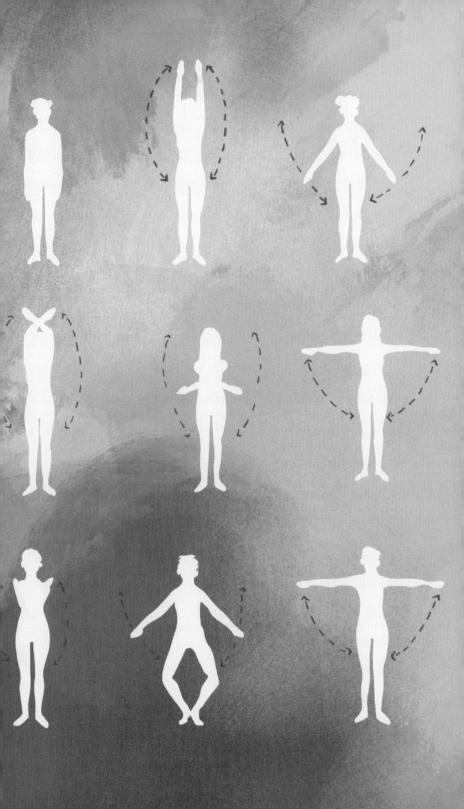

WEIGH IT UP

Free weights v resistance machines

- Strength training can involve free weights or resistance machines. The latter, which tend to target specific muscles and have visual instructions, are a good starting point for beginners. Free weight exercises engage many parts of the body at the same time.

- Free weights also provide more choices over machines. It's wise to do some research in advance as to how to use them safely and effectively, but it's also fine to use your phone if you wish to refer to relevant websites while at the gym.

- A couple of sessions with a fully qualified PT can help to outline your goals and give you the tools and ability to pursue them on your own with personally designed programmes. Do your research and make sure to choose someone whose specialisms match your goals and with whom you feel comfortable to ask questions. Many gym staff will also be happy to share knowledge and tips about how to exercise safely and effectively.

- There are several apps and online videos that demonstrate how to use weights safely – nhs.uk has equipment-free strength and flexibility podcasts available to download. Many gyms also offer free daily or weekly passes, which is a great way to try before you buy.

Home workouts

- If a gym membership isn't suitable, you can still reap the benefits of strength training at home. And this allows for more flexibility so that you can schedule your workout for where and when you want to exercise.

- Body-weight exercises such as squats, push-ups, hip raises, lunges, planks and burpees, are a good choice as they build strength, require no equipment and can be done just about anywhere – at home, in the garden or even in the park with friends.

SAFETY FIRST

- Before working out, ensure you're hydrated and fuelled.
- Remember to stretch both before and after exercising.
- Start with technique, concentration and breathing – they're more important than the weight you lift.
- When you do begin to add weight, start light.
- Test your limits slowly and see what feels comfortable.
- Carry weights with caution.
- Ignore the size of the weights others are using – everyone is different and you only have your own body to go by.
- Keep your breathing steady when lifting.
- Don't assume someone who appears fitter than you has the right posture for the work they're doing. If you know the exercise you are performing is correct, have the confidence to continue as you are.
- Introduce heavier weights gradually over time to challenge yourself without causing damage. You could consult a PT for advice on when is the right time to go heavier.

Please check with your GP before embarking on any exercise programme. Anyone with osteoporosis is advised to seek expert medical advice and use weights under supervision.

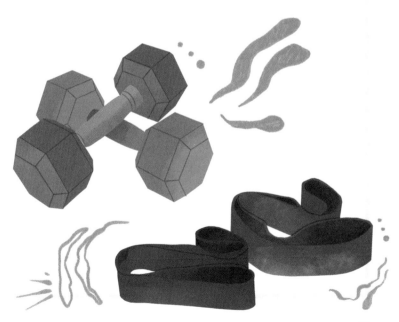

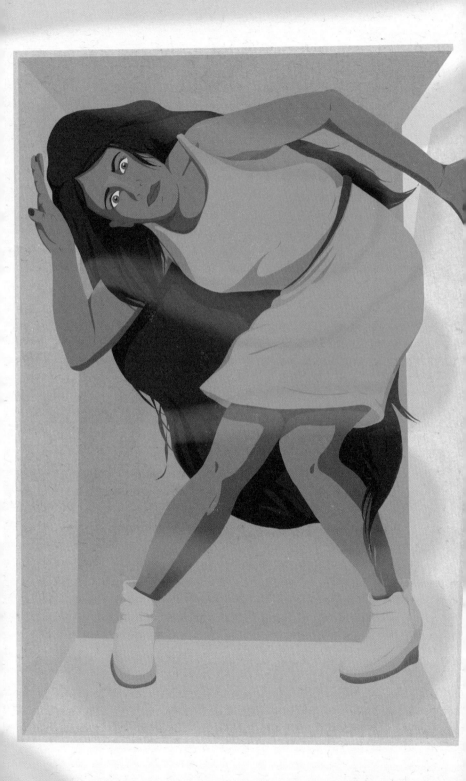

In search of closure

It's easy to feel stuck when ruminating over past events and struggling to find answers as to what happened and why. Here, clinical psychologist Dr Ahona Guha explores some of the ways to help loosen the ties, making it easier to move forward

Tom* sat in my office, nervously frowning at a tissue. He had been referred to me by law-enforcement professionals after being charged with stalking a former partner. 'I just wanted closure,' he pleaded. 'I only wanted to find her so I could talk to her and understand why the relationship ended. She wouldn't speak to me and I couldn't move on without closure.' In this last aspect, Tom isn't alone. In fact, many people voluntarily seek professional help in pursuit of closure after complex events. Whether it's harmful relationships, career pathways that have stagnated, friendships beset by toxicity or bad business decisions, people often find it difficult to understand, heal and move on from difficult episodes in life.

What is meant by closure?

As a term, psychological closure has been embraced by the popular media, usually in the context of the end of romantic relationships. It involves a sense of psychological completion, including cognitively understanding why and how an event occurred, processing it and finding meaning in it.

Historically, the concept of closure derives from the work of a Lithuanian-Soviet cognitive psychologist and psychiatrist, Bluma Zeigarnik. In the 1920s, Bluma discovered that people who were interrupted during a task retained a better memory of the task than those who completed it. From a cognitive perspective, this implies that we have better memory for matters we perceive as incomplete or unfinished than for those we see as completed.

Similarly, a 2010 study found that this also affected how people processed emotions, and that they often regretted and thought more about inaction than about actions they had completed. This seems to suggest that situations left unexplored or somehow incomplete, can weigh heavily on the human mind. Contemplating the 'what-ifs?' is a natural human tendency, but it can also stop people from laying an experience to rest, as it directs focus away from the tasks of closure to ongoing rumination about what happened.

Achieving closure

Closure involves a number of different components: cognitive – how much and how often we think about an event; emotions – how we feel about it; and memories – the recall of that event. Overall, to find closure, it's important to arrive at a helpful understanding of the situation, find a way to create some meaning from it, and allow and process any emotions that might arise.

Forensic psychologist Bonnie Albrecht says: 'Closure is a self-compassionate process – and possibly one that never actually "closes". We can never control what another person will do or how they may change, so closure needs to be focused on the self, and the learnings and growth that one can take from any given situation or event.'

Why do we get stuck?

Sometimes, people become stuck in the process of finding closure. This can happen for several reasons. Some experiences are overwhelmingly distressing and it can be challenging to experience and process all the emotions that have arisen. Situations that involve complicated or intense grief, such as an unexpected bereavement or an especially difficult divorce, can also bring up overpowering feelings and questions to which there might not be any answers. This makes it difficult for people to find cognitive or emotional closure.

There are also occasions when an event feels completely out of a person's control, such as a break-up they didn't instigate or desire. In these circumstances, it's common for people to try to seek answers in order to regain a sense of control. Tom, who we heard from at the start, believed that if he could understand why his partner had left him, he'd be able to convince her to return. Then he could stop feeling hurt and sad. Often, the most challenging events from which to find closure are those that involve being wounded by other people.

Negative and very recent situations are also more likely to remain unprocessed, as are those requiring a leap of faith, such as moving from the comfort of a relationship into the unknown. The latter can bring about anxiety and a desire to remain in the space of the known, which manifest as difficulties with letting go.

It's in your hands

Seeking closure involves a tacit understanding that you might never fully gain the answers you're searching for from others and that it might instead be a gift you need to give to yourself. Finding closure is ultimately an exercise in meaning-making, in determining the meaning and impacts of a difficult experience, understanding how to integrate the experience into your world view and sense of self, and the lessons you need to take away from an experience.

'Closure is an opportunity to identify a self-compassionate and meaningful conclusion to an event,' says Bonnie, 'and then to carry this learning forward to apply to the next chapter of our lives.'

CLOSURE: A THREE-PART PROCESS

When trying to find closure, it's helpful to engage in three main tasks. These are: fully understanding a situation; exploring and expressing the difficult emotions that might have arisen; and allowing time and distance from the event, so it can be viewed as one episode in a life narrative, rather than the sole defining event.

1. Understanding what's happened
It's helpful to spend time thinking about the event in a constructive manner. Instead of aimless rumination, this is targeted thought, which is designed to help explore and learn from a situation. It's important to set some clear parameters around this process, such as reserving an afternoon for it and then wrapping up the time by journalling or writing yourself a letter. Thoughts are focused on trying to learn and grow rather than blaming (self or others), defending or denying the reality (for example, it shouldn't have happened this way).

2. Exploring emotions
The main tasks here involve recognising that a range of difficult feelings might arise and allowing all these emotions to exist. People sometimes try to escape difficult feelings and numb themselves, or engage in intellectualisation as a way of avoiding them. But it's important to attempt to accept the feelings, to sit with them and express them, through crying, talking, drawing or writing, for example. Strong emotions can feel scary, but they can settle with time if expression has been allowed.

3. Creating distance
Allowing time and distance from a painful event is essential. This might involve practical steps, such as moving house or deciding on a period of no contact with an individual. Equally, it might also include allowing and acknowledging pain and remembering that it will usually abate with time. One question to ask yourself might be: 'Will I feel this way in five years' time?' To create closure, it can be helpful to physically contain the experience. Researchers have found that writing about a difficult episode and placing it in a sealed envelope or box can help people process the experience quicker. It's worth considering whether you could engage in a similar task.

CREATE YOUR CLOSURE TOOLKIT

If you have been through a difficult experience and want to find closure, start by asking yourself some questions.

What was the painful event?

....

....

....

....

....

Which parts of the event were most distressing?

....

....

....

....

....

Does it remind you of other times in your life?

....

....

....

....

....

What was your contribution to it?

....

....

....

....

....

....

Which aspects of the situation were influenced by someone else? Which aspects could you control? What was out of your control?

....

....

....

....

....

....

What could you do differently next time?

....

....

....

....

....

....

....

How might you grow through this?

What is one action you can take to let go of what you can't control?

Words for myself

Using the previous closure toolkit questions, explore your feelings in the space here. You might choose to write a letter to yourself or list difficult emotions and how they might be soothed. If desired, you could destroy or bury the words later.

....

....

....

....

....

....

....

....

....

....

....

....

....

....

....

....

....

....

Moments of trust

It can take years to build and be shattered in an instant, but having faith in others, as well as yourself, could save heartache and disappointment

You've probably heard the phrase 'no man is an island'. This aphorism originates in prose by the metaphysical poet John Donne. It continues 'every man is a piece of the continent, a part of the main'. Even though times have moved on since 1624, when Donne wrote those words, the sentiment remains the same: you're part of something bigger than yourself. If that's true, what makes you so connected?

Arguably, one of the most important elements of a friendship is trust. It's also central to romantic relationships, healthcare, the workplace and business transactions. It's even necessary for a sense of self-worth. Would you bank with a company if you thought it was untrustworthy? Would you leave your pet with a friend you knew to be irresponsible? Trust relies on being sure the other person in any transaction or relationship is honest and will do the right thing by you. When it's shaken, it can make human relations difficult, or even risky. But what exactly is this elusive concept?

Trust versus reliance

Some believe trust and reliance are one and the same. After all, they share many features. You might rely on the goodwill of a stranger, and hope they return a lost purse. You might trust a friend to give constructive advice about a relationship problem. Both trust and reliance are integral to helping relationships to flourish and form the backbone of many social interactions. What would be the point of going to school if you couldn't believe what the teachers told you? What sense would it make to visit your GP if you couldn't rely on their advice?

The two concepts are different, however. Throughout time, societies and cultures worldwide have had different words for trust that have had varying meanings, whereas reliance tends to have one word to express one specific thing. The two also provoke different responses. Feelings of misplaced reliance often relate to less intense emotions, which tend to be self-directed ('I was wrong to rely on you', for example). Misplaced trust, on the other hand, frequently relates to more extreme emotions, such as betrayal ('I trusted you, and you hurt me'). Philosopher Annette Baier wrote that 'trusting can be betrayed, or at least let down, and not just disappointed'.

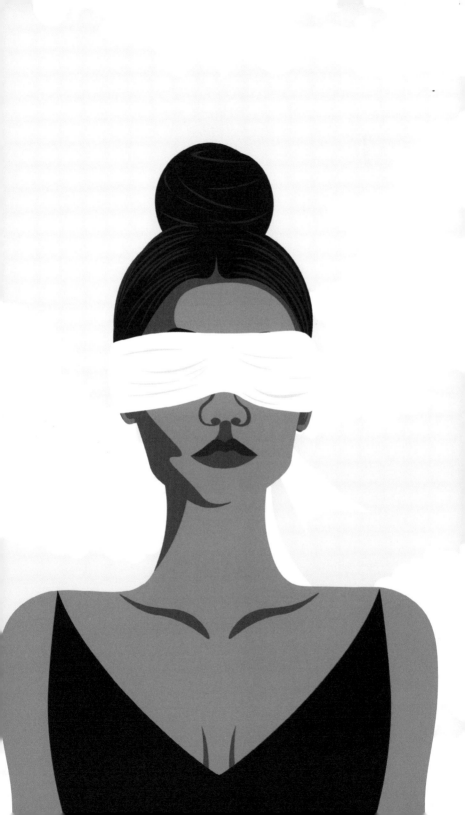

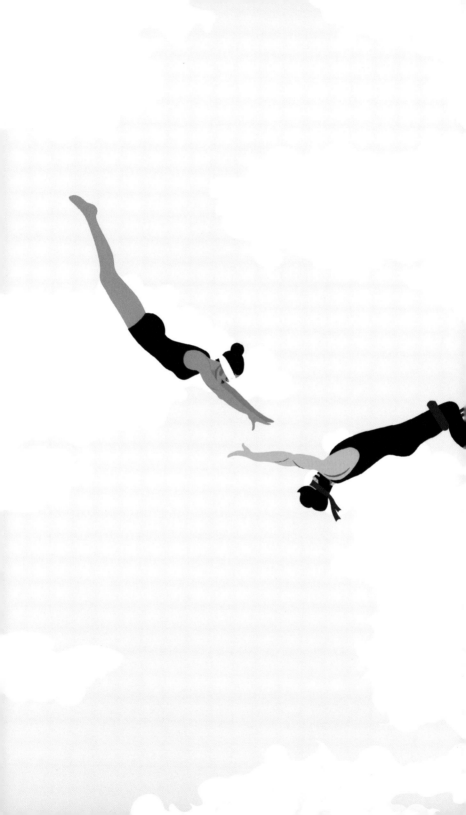

Something extra

Imagine this scenario: you have confidence in a friend, so you decide to ask them to look after your dog while you go to the shops. This belief in them might come from having witnessed their compassion towards a grief-stricken pal and seen their organisational ability in juggling work deadlines with family commitments. The two factors might make them appear the perfect candidate for dog-sitting. Philosopher Nancy Nyquist Potter agrees with this thinking. She defines a trustworthy person as someone 'who can be counted on, as a matter of the sort of person he or she is'.

Conversely, you might rely on someone to act badly. You've probably seen compulsive liars on TV, such as Creed Bratton in the US version of *The Office*. His colleagues could pretty much depend on him to invent a fabrication, but would they trust him to lie? Many philosophers say that trust is a kind of reliance but not mere reliance – because it involves an extra factor. They say this is something like goodwill or benevolence – in other words, you trust someone to act well.

Commitment and risk

Sometimes it's useful to think about things from another angle. Philosopher Katherine Hawley believed trust was akin to commitment in a relationship. So, when you have faith in someone, you ask them to pledge themselves to do something for you, such as helping with the weekly shopping. She pointed out that such commitment involved risk, which was part and parcel as to why the process could seem unnerving. Anyone who's ever loaned a friend a much-loved item and been baffled when it wasn't returned will recognise the concern. And it's not just property that can be lost. In some cases, the friendship itself slowly starts to fade.

The good news is you can determine the process. One way to think about trust is as a two-way system – you can exert control over what you entrust and to whom. You might want to think about trusting wisely. What does that look like? You could, for example, weigh up previous evidence of trustworthiness before lending someone a sentimental or expensive-to-replace item. What that evidence looks like will depend on the relationship. One place to start might be to explore a friend's transparency. If you've asked them to dog-sit, for example, would they be likely to give you notice if their plans changed and they were no longer able to help? Or would they stay schtum and let you down at the last minute?

Find the right fit

Of course, everyone has different strengths. One person might be a great listener, another an intuitive problem-solver and a third a true negotiator. Compiling lists of the most trustworthy friends, however, isn't necessarily the answer. You could instead ask yourself who's the most appropriate or well-qualified friend for a particular job. You wouldn't, for example, depend on a car mechanic to repair your shoes, or a cobbler to fix an engine. Similarly, you'd be more likely to ask a feline-loving friend to cat-sit than you would someone who had a serious aversion to all creatures with claws.

New friendships

All these decisions, of course, are easier to make when you have evidence of previous behaviour to fall back on. But how do you begin to have faith in a new friend? That can be challenging, as clinical psychologist Tamara Scully explains: 'Trust is fundamental to strong positive relationships but it's not something that is there immediately.'

In this case, it can help to start small and work your way up. You could lend a new acquaintance a well-read book or much-watched DVD that you don't mind losing, especially if it fits their interests. This will give you an idea as to whether it will be returned. It's important, however, to keep it natural and not force the issue. If, for example, they're going through trying times but choose to be around close family rather than new friends, don't take it personally. As Tamara says: 'Trust is something you build together in small moments of interaction – keeping promises, supporting one another, showing up, apologising if you get something wrong.'

Earned, not given

Once you begin to count on one another, you could impart something that holds more personal value, such as a favourite recipe book. For some there might be a temptation to buy expensive new items with the intention of lending them, but try to remember that trust can't be bought.

In the words of American businessman Max de Pree: 'Earning trust is not easy, nor is it cheap, nor does it happen quickly. Earning trust is hard and demanding work. Trust comes only with genuine effort, never with a lick and a promise.' Sometimes things fall apart, and you might put your faith in someone who lets you down. Trusting again might feel frightening, but ultimately, it's the bridge that connects islands.

TRUSTING YOURSELF

Are you a trustworthy person? If you believe the answer is no, you might be failing to perceive yourself as others see you. Here are some pointers to bear in mind:

1. Take time out

Asserting yourself is a step on the path to trusting yourself. Everyone needs time to rest. You don't have to be constantly on call for other people. Of course, if you're in a care-giving role, it might be difficult to get time to yourself, but everyone would benefit from stopping at some point in the day, even if only for five minutes.

My favourite ways to make time for myself...

....

....

....

....

....

....

....

....

....

....

....

....

....

....

....

2. Be honest

Try to be candid if friends or family have asked you to take on too much. Of course, it's important to stay polite. If you're struggling to find the words, you could say something like: 'I've got a lot on my plate at work at the moment. Is it okay if you get someone else to dog-sit?' Recognising your needs also means you'll be more attentive to the needs of others.

Things I'd rather say no to...

....

....

....

....

....

....

....

....

....

....

....

....

....

....

....

....

3. Follow your goals

Whatever the size or the nature of any intentions you've set for yourself, follow them up. So, if you've decided to read more, put your feet up and go for it; if you want to learn the piano, set aside time to practise; if you're trying to master a new language, get talking. Schedule the time in your diary.

Goals and activities I want to commit to...

....

....

....

....

....

....

....

....

....

....

....

....

....

....

....

....

....

4. Forgive yourself

It's okay to make mistakes. If a friend trusted you with her expensive camera and you've lost or broken it, don't beat yourself up about it. Instead, be transparent and as upfront about it as soon as possible.

My apology letter...

....

....

....

....

....

....

....

....

....

....

....

....

....

....

....

....

....

5. Believe in yourself

It might be tempting to see rough patches as proof that you can't be trusted. This isn't true. Every time you return after a setback is more evidence that you can weather a storm. Whatever that looks like for you, be it a challenging presentation at work or bravely facing a situation that causes personal anxiety, it reflects your character as a person upon whom others can rely and trust.

My proudest moments...

....

....

....

....

....

....

....

....

....

....

....

....

....

....

....

If you find that issues of trust are affecting your ability to make friends and maintain relationships, and you'd like to change the situation, it might help to talk to your GP or a counsellor. There are also many online groups and charities that can help, including mind.org.uk.

Curb the chaos

Chaotic thinking can bring inspired ideas, but also lead to confusion and a strong sense of being overwhelmed. There are, however, ways to moderate the negatives of a mind under stress

If you've ever felt your mind was brimming over with random thoughts, like an Instagram feed that's scrolling too fast for your eyes to focus on anything, you might have been experiencing chaotic thinking. Sometimes this hectic flash of ideas can bring creative inspiration or cause a switch into superpower mode, but if you feel you're in a battle with your own brain, especially when those thoughts come thick and fast, it can be stressful too. Here, US-based marriage and family therapist Elizabeth Hinkle explains chaotic thinking and shares her guidance on how to help curb the confusion it can bring.

What is chaotic thinking?
'It describes types of thoughts that flood your brain very quickly. They can feel intense and overwhelming, and they don't always make sense. These chaotic thoughts usually feel disorganised, out of place and impulsive.'

What's the difference between chaotic and manic thinking?
'Chaos and mania are different beasts that manifest in various ways. Chaos would typically be how you're responding to a particular stressful situation. For example, you might be clashing with a partner, which could lead to a barrage of thoughts like: "I can't take this any more" or "I don't know what to do" and "Why do we fight so much?"

'A manic episode comes from a chemical/biological response in the brain and isn't usually triggered by an outside event. It often includes irrational thoughts or ones that inflate reality, for example, thinking something like: "Nothing could hurt me right now, I am invincible." In extreme cases, mania involves impulsive and/or risk-taking behaviour that's out of character for that person.'

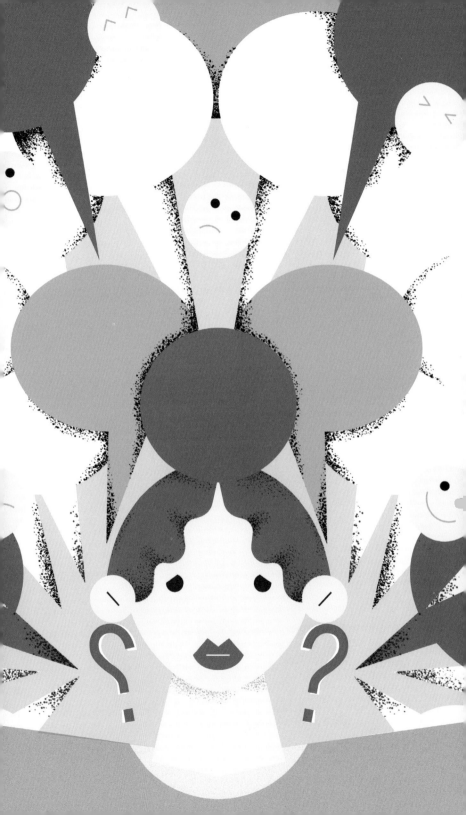

What makes a chaotic episode worse?

'Stress can make any type of thinking more chaotic and difficult. When we're stressed, we tend not to breathe as slowly or deeply. This can lead to reduced oxygen levels, which makes it harder to think clearly. It also creates anxious feelings that interfere with thought clarity and focus. Both chaotic and manic episodes could happen regardless of lifestyle choices or personality traits. However, a habit such as substance misuse could contribute to triggering or worsening an episode.'

Is feeling this way always negative, or can it be put to good use?

'It's rare that something happening is either solely good or bad. It seems much of this is about each person and what works for them. If your thoughts are bothering you, it's good to reach out and talk to a trusted family member or a friend and/or a professional when that's needed. If your thoughts help you to be more creative and it doesn't feel harmful, though, that's great.'

What types of therapy can help to calm chaotic thinking?

According to Talkspace, an online therapy website to which Elizabeth contributes, there are more than 50 types of therapeutic approaches, but some focus specifically on how people think. 'Cognitive behavioural therapy is the main one. It helps people recognise those automatic and distorted types of thoughts, such as assumptions, and encourages them to think differently to encourage a different emotion.

'If, for example, someone hasn't responded to your text and the thought "they must hate me" crosses your mind, it's helpful to focus on the facts. Something like: "I don't know why she hasn't replied. She could be busy right now. It might not have anything to do with me." Usually a person will feel less upset if they practise techniques like this.'

When should you ask for help?

'If you notice thoughts are disturbing you on a regular basis, it could be a sign it's a good time to seek professional help. Reach out immediately if you are having thoughts of hurting yourself or someone else.'

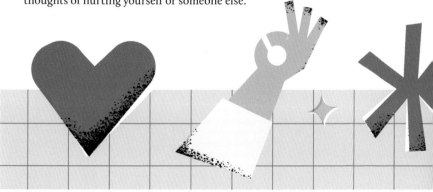

FINDING CALM

How to move past difficult thinking to a calmer place.

1. Identify
Work out how you're feeling and clarify the emotion you're experiencing. Is it sadness, anger, hurt, confusion?

2. Understand
Unpick what has contributed to your feeling this way and any potential triggers that might have been responsible for it.

3. Recognise
Once you're aware of how you feel and why, look again at your emotions. As Elizabeth emphasises, feelings aren't right or wrong, good or bad, they are what they are. You aren't agreeing or disagreeing with the emotion, you are recognising it.

4. Reframe
Remind yourself that emotions come and go. Stick to the facts and find a mantra you find calming. Try reframing your thoughts to ones that are more helpful to you – and seek professional help with this if needed.

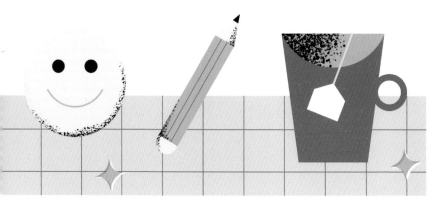

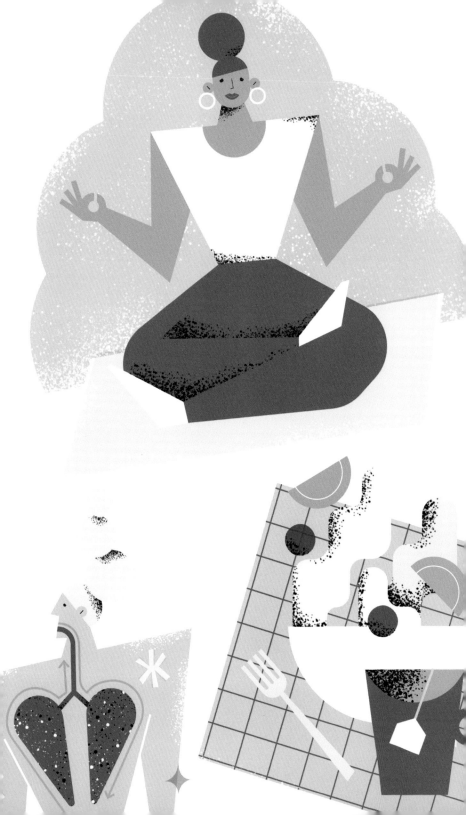

SLOW IT DOWN

Active ways to help tame chaotic thoughts.

- Move your body. Walking, stretching, yoga, jogging, or even just dancing around your kitchen, could help.

- Check your fluid intake and nutrition. The NHS Eatwell Guide (nhs.uk) recommends drinking six to eight glasses of fluid daily – besides water, lower-fat milk, tea and coffee count – and having at least five portions of a variety of fruit and veg a day. Also make sure you're eating at regular intervals.

- Put pen to paper. Write down your chaotic thoughts if you can, as it might help to process them later.

- Open up. Talk to a friend or a family member, or reach out for help from a professional therapist.

- Take deep, slow breaths. Inhale through your nose and out through your mouth for a few minutes to improve oxygen intake. If things don't improve, give the exercise over the page a try.

If you're experiencing a mental health crisis and need immediate help, the following organisations all offer free and confidential advice and support 24/7: samaritans.org, giveusashout.org, crisistextline.org.

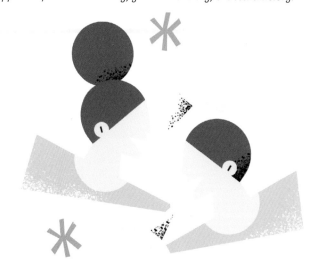

Bubble vision

*How an imaginary personal sphere can form
a perfect protective shield*

Staying calm and resilient when facing life's stresses and strains can be a challenge. Many people start the day full of inner strength only to feel it draining away when confronted with external pressures. These could be anything from receiving criticism to absorbing a friend's sadness or hearing an upsetting story on the news.

Feeling shaken by outside events or emotions is especially common for those who are sensitive to the moods or energy of others, or who find maintaining boundaries difficult. But scientific studies show that visualisation exercises are an effective way to increase resilience. Picturing a comforting image leads to the release of the same mood-boosting chemicals in the brain as the imagined scene would produce in real life.

One way of creating a sanctuary for yourself is to build an imaginary protective bubble. Visualising this can generate a sense of safety and security that you can call on in any potentially unsettling scenario.

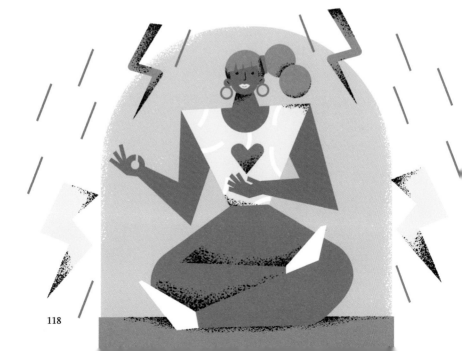

BUILD YOUR BUBBLE

- Standing or sitting in an upright chair, breathe in slowly to the count of three. Then exhale gently to the count of five, breathing out any worries or negative thoughts and relaxing your muscles.

- Feel the way your feet are rooted to the ground and stretch your arms up above your head, with your palms facing upwards.

- Keeping your arms stretched out to each side, lower your hands slowly and visualise a shimmering bubble flowing out around you from the tips of your fingers.

- Lower your arms until they come to rest against your body, sending the edges of the bubble downwards in your mind until it's beneath the soles of your feet, where it's then sealed.

- Take another deep breath in and, as you inhale this time, visualise a radiant golden light travelling up through your feet from deep in the ground beneath and filling your whole body.

- As you exhale, imagine your breath billowing out and filling the bubble with this powerful golden light to form a force field around you.

- Observe how any negative energy that heads towards you from outside just gently bounces off the smooth, reflective surface of the bubble.

- Notice how secure you feel in this protective dome and know that, whatever comes your way, you're safe inside. With regular practice of the visualisation, this sense of security can become second nature.

'Mental health: having enough safe places in your mind for your thoughts to settle'

Alain de Botton

All shapes and sizes

Families are as complex as the individuals that make them up, yet the view of these inherited groups is often singular, that they're identikit units and the be-all and end-all of everything. Is there room for a more nuanced story?

Family is important. It's the first social group we belong to. Much is learned from this early unit – irrespective of its composition or boundaries – including role responsibilities, boundaries and how to negotiate with others. However, with age comes the freedom to create our own milieu.

Finding your place

I don't have a problem with family, many of my best times have been spent with my parents and cousins. In fact, as I sit and write these words, the days that I hanker for most are the simplest ones that involve drinking tea and eating cake with my mother and gran. But since they both passed, my family has somewhat dispersed. What once was is no more. I have found myself in an amorphous group connected by blood. And this group, comprising aunts, uncles and cousins, often does not represent me. Some of them do, as individuals, but not as the collective known as the Family.

Since some key members passed away, I've grappled with the idea of belonging. Family isn't fixed, of course, members will die and new ones will be born. It's the natural pruning of the family tree, not unlike the deadheading of a rose bush. So it stands to reason that a unit that once provided a sense of belonging or was comfortable might no longer feel like home. This all sounds rather logical and obvious, but it's a sentiment that's often followed by a societal pearl-clutching.

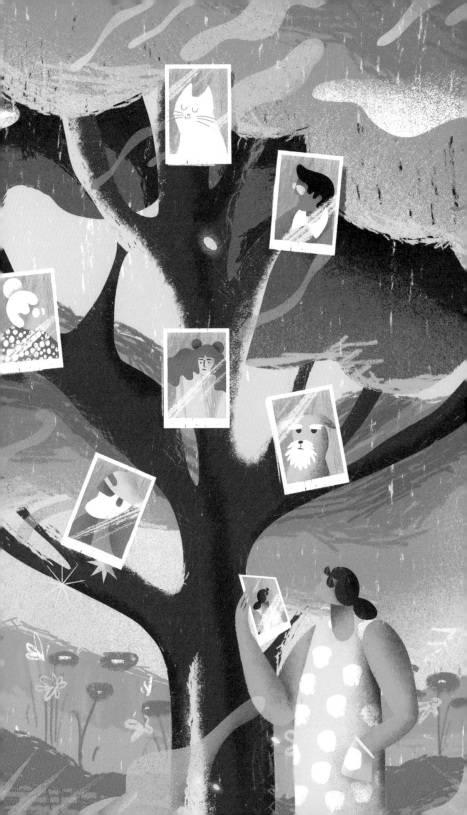

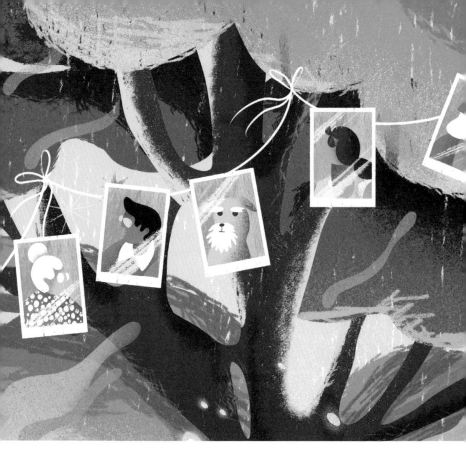

Mixed feelings

The statement that 'family is all that matters' expresses nothing more than an ideal. And while it's often true, like everything in life, it's mutable. For those who find they're more suitably fitted in other groups, with friends for example, the statement might suggest they've failed or that their feeling of misplacement among the people with whom they grew up or those who raised them is down to their inadequacy. But families are as individual as the people who make them up. An article I read about the importance of this unit stated that family never fails you. But that's only one version, and my experience is to the contrary. The concern, however, is that sticking to this one mantra risks telling half-truths.

'Whatever your secret, live your own truth; life is too short'

Oprah Winfrey

Another truth

Arguably, if society was more honest about the spectrum of experiences individuals face with their own, people whose families don't fit them would feel less like failures. Yet there seems to be only one narrative. There's much written and said on the merits of keeping close those who are related to us, but little about how these relationships, like any other, can sour. Divorces and friendship breakdowns are frequently and publicly unpicked, but family relationships rarely come under the same microscope. And because of this, when people have asked me about mine, I've sometimes pretended it's a perfectly functioning unit.

Telling the truth, that I'm estranged from some relatives, provokes bewilderment and judgment: 'But that's your sister/brother/aunt,' comes the reply, suggesting that relations have a licence to treat us however they wish, badly or otherwise. It also implies that we're obliged to forgive pernicious treatment at the hands of family members. The response often betrays an unwillingness to accept that sometimes these close relationships can and do break down beyond repair. And this attitude silences people like me.

I've often wondered, however, if my lack of honesty helps to perpetuate the myth that families can do no wrong. So, at times, when I feel I'm in safe company, I try to tell the truth. And surprisingly, it doesn't always garner the same disbelieving response with which I'm so familiar. In fact, many people have experienced similar family strife. Perhaps, contrary to the popular belief that 'family is all that matters', it might be closer to the truth and more of a universal experience to say 'family matters, sometimes'.

Moving on

Even with my earlier declaration that my most cherished memories involve family, it's not a contradiction to say this. All relationships are subject to change. It takes courage to walk away from something that no longer serves you well. Change is both inevitable and essential in life. It's folly to hang on to something that once was but no longer is. It takes insight and, albeit painful, acknowledgement to know the difference. It can be a freeing revelation that allows you to paint and structure your own life. I have many homes and have lived many lives from acknowledging that family is not always the one that raises you.

UNPICKING THE TIES

- Most people have family issues, so don't feel embarrassed if your unit isn't perfect.

- Not everyone needs to know your life story. If you don't feel comfortable telling someone about your situation, don't.

- Don't feel bad if you pick and choose who you want to spend your time with. Most people don't get on with everyone, and that's normal.

- You can build your own hand-picked family, made up of friends and relations that become a supportive unit that's more reflective of you.

- Stop comparing your family with others. Yes, some are great, but most people don't openly discuss the difficulties within their unit. As the saying goes: 'You don't know what happens behind closed doors.'

- Don't let anyone ever tell you friends can't be family. They can. In fact, they can be at the heart of better relationships because you've chosen them.

- Accept your situation. It takes courage to look at things with clarity. If members of your family have hurt you more than they've shown you love, then it's okay to distance yourself. You don't need to cut them off, just limit your time with them.

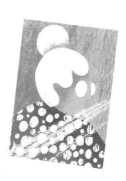

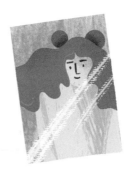

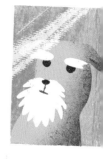

UNDERSTANDING YOUR FAMILY

1. When you think about your relationships, it can be helpful to consider the following:

When you're together, how do they make you feel?

....

....

....

....

....

....

....

....

Do you feel cared for and supported?

....

....

....

....

....

....

....

Have you ever made them aware of these feelings?

....

....

....

....

....

....

....

....

Do you try to show up for them the way you wish they did for you?

....

....

....

....

....

....

....

....

2. Try examining your relationship with individual family members using the prompts below:

I feel like I can be myself around...

....

....

....

I feel energised after spending time with...

....

....

....

I think my relationship needs to change with...

....

....

....

Things that are missing from this relationship are...

....

....

....

Realising that a relationship needs to change can be difficult, but asking for what you want and need shows you care enough to do something about it. In certain instances, setting boundaries with someone can make a relationship stronger. However, if someone in your family is not good for your mental health, don't feel obliged to continue the relationship. Understandably, some ties are easier to end than others, but there are organisations that can help, including the charity Stand Alone, which helps people deal with family estrangement.

Breathe

BREATHE is a trademark of Guild of Master Craftsman Publications Ltd

First published 2023 by
Ammonite Press
an imprint of Guild of Master Craftsman Publications Ltd
Castle Place, 166 High Street, Lewes, East Sussex BN7 1XU, United Kingdom

www.ammonitepress.com
www.breathemagazine.com

Compiled by Susie Duff
Editorial: Catherine Kielthy, Jane Roe, Josie Fletcher
Words credits: Jade Beecroft, Regina A Bernard, PhD, Lizzie Bestow, Claire Blackmore, Judy Cogan, Kerry Dolan, Yvonne Gavan, Ahona Guha, Stephanie Lam, Leah Larwood, Caroline Pattenden, Chloe Rhodes, Kiran Sidhu

Illustrations: Carolina Altavilla, Magda Azab, Amy Leonard, Irina Perju, Silvia Stecher, Maggie Stephenson, Michelle Urra
Cover illustration: Maggie Stephenson

ISBN 978 1 78145 482 4

Breathe Magazine
Publisher: Jonathan Grogan

Colour reproduction by GMC Reprographics
Printed and bound in China

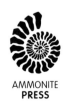

AMMONITE
PRESS